OXFORD PAIN MANAGEMENT LIBRARY

Migraine and other Primary Headaches

OPML

OXFORD PAIN MANAGEMENT LIBRARY

Migraine and other Primary Headaches

Edited by

Dr Anne MacGregor

Honorary Director of Clinical Research,
The City of London Migraine Clinic,
London, UK

Professor Rigmor Jensen

Danish Headache Center,
Department of Neurology,
Glostrup Hospital,
University of Copenhagen,
Glostrup, Denmark

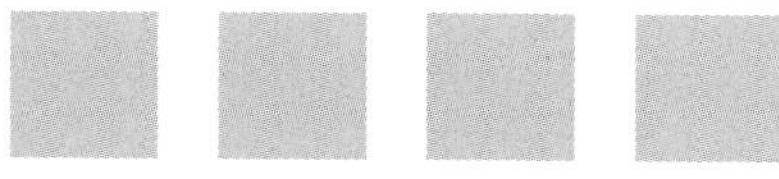

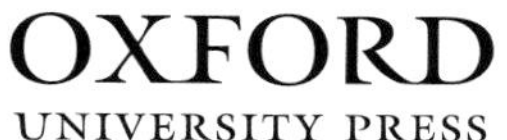

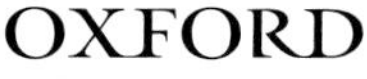

Great Clarendon Street, Oxford OX2 6DP

Oxford University Press is a department of the University of Oxford.
It furthers the University's objective of excellence in research, scholarship, and education by publishing worldwide in

Oxford New York

Auckland Cape Town Dar es Salaam Hong Kong Karachi
Kuala Lumpur Madrid Melbourne Mexico City Nairobi
New Delhi Shanghai Taipei Toronto

With offices in

Argentina Austria Brazil Chile Czech Republic France Greece
Guatemala Hungary Italy Japan Poland Portugal Singapore
South Korea Switzerland Thailand Turkey Ukraine Vietnam

Oxford is a registered trade mark of Oxford University Press in the UK and in certain other countries

Published in the United States
by Oxford University Press Inc., New York

First published 2008

British Library Cataloguing in Publication Data

Data available

Library of Congress Cataloging in Publication Data

Data available

Typeset by Newgen Imaging Systems (P) Ltd, Chennai, India
Printed in Italy
on acid-free paper by
L.E.G.O. S.p.A - Lavis (TN)

ISBN 978–0–19–954514–8

10 9 8 7 6 5 4 3 2 1

Contents

Preface

We are delighted to have had the opportunity to collaborate with key headache specialists in Europe to present this text. Although the title of the book suggests a focus on migraine and other primary headaches, the text would not be complete without a review of the consequences of mismanagement of primary headaches, i.e. medication overuse headache, or misdiagnosis of primary headache in the presentation of a secondary headache disorder.

We have chosen to separate each headache into sections on diagnosis, pathophysiology, and management, an approach which has enabled us to introduce a broad spectrum of views from opinion leaders who, ultimately, share the same wish to provide a better level of care for patients with headache. As editors, it has been our pleasure to have the opportunity to work with our expert colleagues, each of whom has provided an easy to read but comprehensive overview of their specialist subject.

It has been both a privilege and an education to edit this work and we hope that our readers will enjoy a similar experience, benefiting from the individual and collective expertise of the authors.

Anne MacGregor and Rigmor Jensen, July 2008

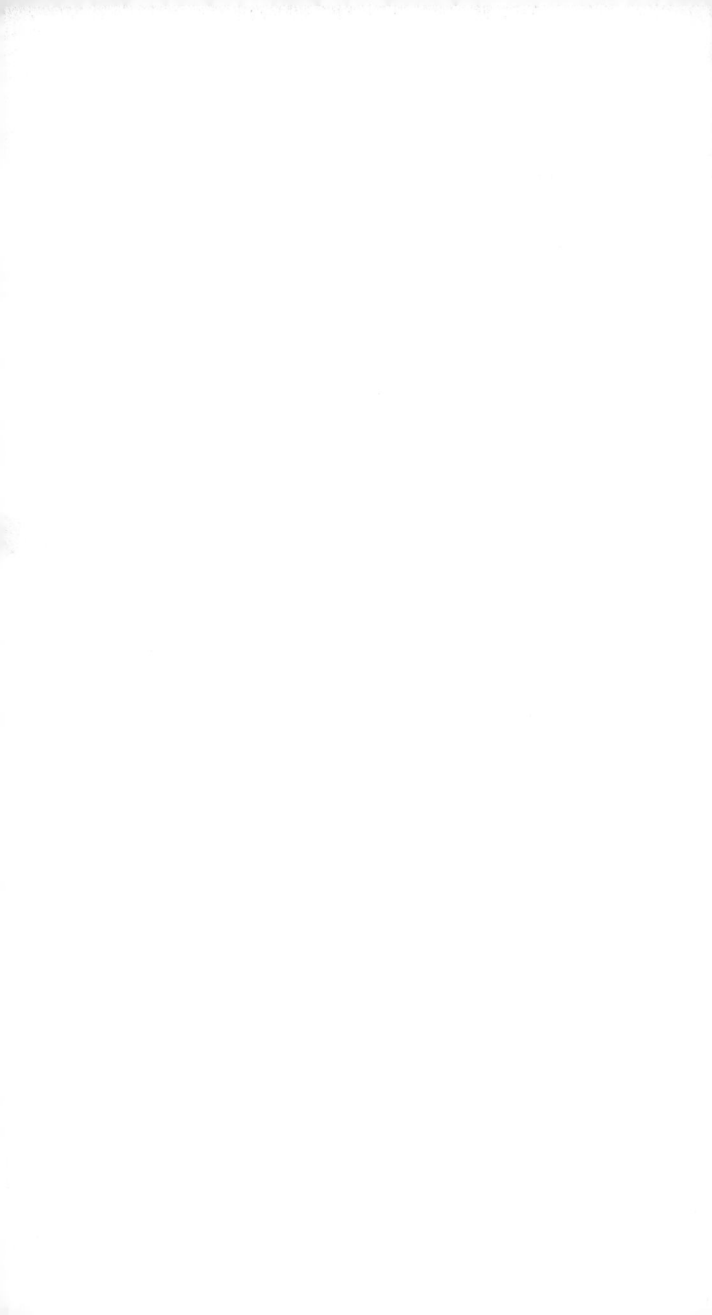

Symbols and abbreviations

💣	Bomb (controversial topic)
ATPase	adenosine triphosphatase
BI	brainstem interneurone
BOLD	blood oxygen level-dependent
CBT	cognitive behavioural therapy
CCH	chronic cluster headache
CGRP	calcitonin gene-related peptide
CI	confidence interval
CH	cluster headache
CPH	chronic paroxysmal hemicrania
CRGP	calcitonin gene-related peptide
CSD	cortical spreading depression
CSF	cerebrospinal fluid
CT	computed tomography
CTTH	chronic tension-type headache
CVT	cerebral venous thrombosis
ECG	electrocardiography
ECH	episodic cluster headache
EMG	electromyography
EPH	episodic paroxysmal hemicrania
5-HT	serotonin (5-hydroxytryptamine)
FHM	familial hemiplegic migraine
Ggl	ganglion
GON	greater occipital nerve
GTN	glyceryl trinitrate
HaNDL	syndrome of headache and neurological deficits with CSF lymphocytosis
HC	hemicrania continua
HT	hypothalamus
ICA	internal carotid artery
iNOS	inducible nitric oxide synthase

L-NMMA	N^{G}-monomethyl-L-arginine
LTM	low-threshold mechanosensitive
MA	migraine with aura
MN	motor nuclei
MO	migraine without aura
MRI	magnetic resonance imaging
MRV	magnetic resonance venography
nNOS	neuronal nitric oxide synthase
NO	nitric oxide
NOS	nitric oxide synthase
NSAID	non-steroidal anti-inflammatory drug
PET	positron emission tomography
PH	paroxysmal hemicrania
PMT	pericranial myofascial tissue
PPT	pressure pain threshold
PPT	pterygopalatine
rCBF	regional cerebral blood flow
SAH	subarachnoid haemorrhage
SCG	superior cervical ganglion
SH/TNC	spinal horn and trigeminal nucleus caudalis
SN	suprachiasmatic nucleus
SPECT	single-photon emission computed tomography
SSN	superior salivatory nucleus
SSRI	selective serotonin-reuptake inhibitor
SUNA	short-lasting unilateral neuralgiform headache attacks with cranial autonomic symptoms
SUNCT	short-lasting unilateral neuralgiform headache attacks with conjunctival injection and tearing
TAC	trigeminal autonomic cephalalgia
TIA	transient ischaemic attack
TN	trigeminal neuralgia
TNC	trigeminocervical complex
TTH	tension-type headache
TTS	total tenderness score
WHO	World Health Organization

Contributors

Dr Messoud Ashina
Danish Headache Center, Department of Neurology, Glostrup Hospital, University of Copenhagen,Glostrup, Denmark

Dr Lars Bendtsen
Danish Headache Center, Department of Neurology, Glostrup Hospital, University of Copenhagen, Glostrup, Denmark

Dr Gennaro Bussone
Head of Clinical Neurosciences Department, C. Besta National Neurological Institute, Milan, Italy

Dr Anna S Cohen
National Hospital for Neurology & Neurosurgery, London, UK

Dr Carl Dahlöf
Gothenburg Migraine Clinic, Gothenburg, Sweden

Dr Hans-Christoph Diener
Department of Neurology, University Duisburg-Essen, Germany

Dr Arnaud Fumal
University Department of Neurology, CHR Citadelle Hospital, Liège, Belgium

Professor Rigmor Jensen
Danish Headache Center, Department of Neurology, Glostrup Hospital, University of Copenhagen, Glostrup, Denmark

Dr Zaza Katsarava
Department of Neurology, University Hospital of Essen, Essen, Germany

Dr Massimo Leone
Department of Neurology and Headache Centre, Istituto Nazionale Neurologico, Milano, Italy

Dr Anne MacGregor
Honorary Director of Clinical Research, The City of London Migraine Clinic, London, UK

Dr Arne May
Department of Systems Neuroscience, University Hospital Hamburg Eppendorf, Germany

Dr Jes Olesen
Danish Headache Center, Department of Neurology, Glostrup Hospital, University of Copenhagen,Glostrup, Denmark

Dr Julio Pascual
Chairman of the Department of Neurology, University Hospital, Salamanca, Spain

Dr Kasja Rabe
Department of Neurology, University Hospital of Essen, Essen, Germany

Dr Jean Schoenen
University Department of Neurology, CHR Citadelle Hospital, Liège, Belgium

Introduction

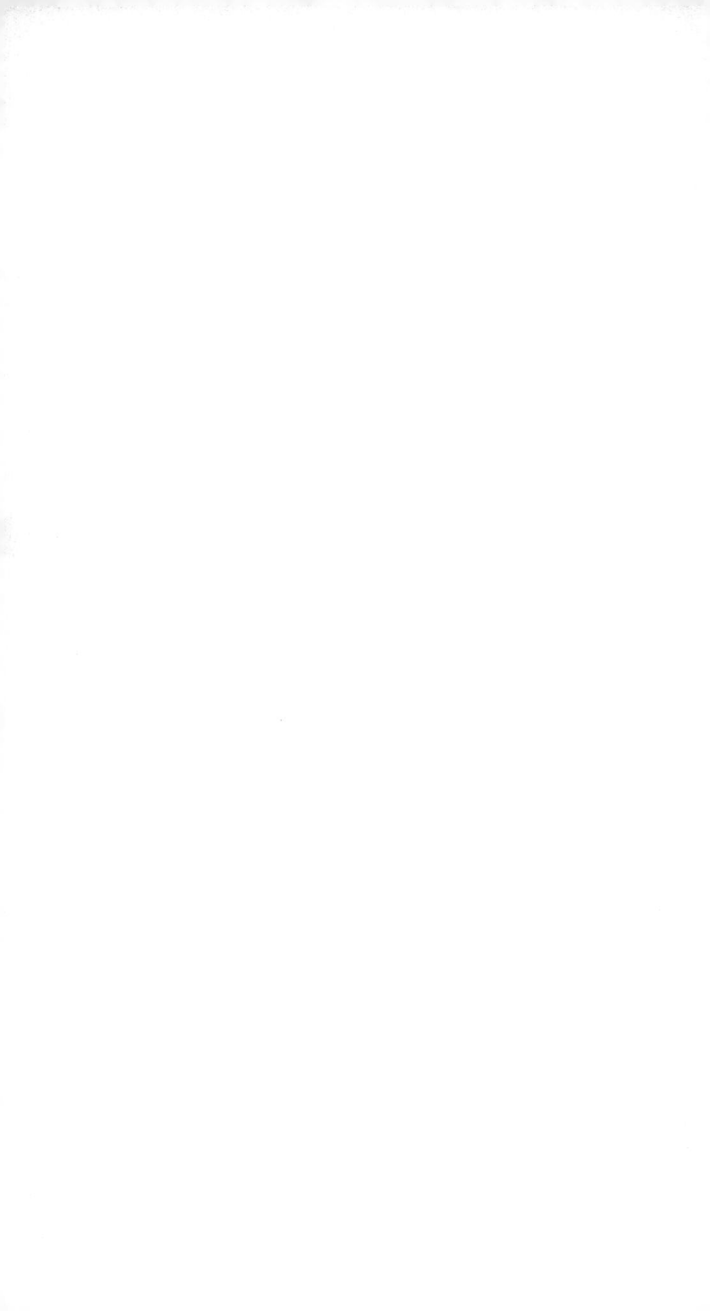

Chapter 1

Headache as a major health problem

Jes Olesen

Key points

- There are more than 100 different kinds of headache that are clearly classified and defined in the International Classification of Headache Disorders.
- A proper headache diagnosis is essential for patient management.
- Distinction is made between primary headaches, which are independent diseases, and secondary headaches, which are caused by another disease.
- Among the primary headaches, migraine is the most important because of a 10% prevalence combined with severe intensity.
- Migraine is among the 20 most burdensome diseases according to the World Health Organization.
- Migraine costs European society 27 000 million euros per year, mostly due to lost working time.
- Non-migraine headaches are estimated to cost an equal or even greater amount, but their impact has been poorly described.
- Headache is the most common reason for consultation in neurological specialist practice and a common problem in general practice.

1.1 Headache classification

Headache disorders were poorly classified and defined until 1988. At that time, the International Headache Society published its International Classification of Headache Disorders (ICHD-1) in which headaches were classified into 13 major groups. The second edition of this classification (ICHD-2) appeared in 2004 and expanded the number of groups to 14 (Box 1.1). There are four groups of primary headache disorder: migraine, tension-type headache, trigeminal autonomic cephalalgias, and other primary headaches. The secondary headaches are classified into eight different groups, cranial neuralgias in one group, and a last group contains disorders that do not fit any of the diagnostic criteria. The classification is hierarchical, using up to 4 digits. As an example, the classification of migraine is given in Box 1.2.

For each disorder, explicit diagnostic criteria are provided. As an example, the diagnostic criteria for frequent episodic tension-type headache are given in Box 3.1. Note that, in order to fulfil the criteria, all the letter headings A, B, C, etc. must be fulfilled. Note also that some criteria are met by fulfilling only two out of four characteristics. The diagnostic criteria are very useful for the clinician because they contain exactly what needs to be obtained from the patient while taking the history. The full classification, as well as an abbreviated pocket-type version, can be found on the website of the International Headache Society: http://www.i-h-s.org. A searchable electronic version in English, German, and Italian can also be found there.

Box 1.1 ICHD-2: major classification groups

1. Migraine
2. Tension-type headache
3. Cluster headache and other trigeminal autonomic cephalalgias
4. Other primary headaches
5. Headache attributed to head and/or neck trauma
6. Headache attributed to cranial or cervical vascular disorder
7. Headache attributed to non-vascular intracranial disorder
8. Headache attributed to a substance or its withdrawal
9. Headache attributed to infection
10. Headache attributed to disorder of homoeostasis
11. Headache or facial pain attributed to disorder of cranium, neck, eyes, ears, nose, sinuses, teeth, mouth, or other facial or cranial structures
12. Headaches attributed to psychiatric disorder
13. Cranial neuralgias and central causes of facial pain
14. Other headache, cranial neuralgia, central or primary facial pain

Box 1.2 Classification of migraine

1	[G43]	Migraine
1.1	[G43.0]	Migraine without aura
1.2	[G43.1]	Migraine with aura
1.2.1	[G43.10]	Typical aura with migraine headache
1.2.2	[G43.10]	Typical aura with non-migraine headache
1.2.3	[G43.104]	Typical aura without headache
1.2.4	[G43.105]	Familial hemiplegic migraine (FHM)
1.2.5	[G43.105]	Sporadic hemiplegic migraine
1.2.6	[G43.103]	Basilar-type migraine
1.3	[G43.82]	Childhood periodic syndromes that are commonly precursors of migraine
1.3.1	[G43.82]	Cyclical vomiting
1.3.2	[G43.820]	Abdominal migraine
1.3.3	[G43.821]	Benign paroxysmal vertigo of childhood
1.4	[G43.81]	Retinal migraine
1.5	[G43.3]	Complications of migraine
1.5.1	[G43.3]	Chronic migraine
1.5.2	[G43.2]	Status migrainosus
1.5.3	[G43.3]	Persistent aura without infarction
1.5.4	[G43.3]	Migrainous infarction
1.5.5	[G43.3] + [G40.x or G41.x]*	Migraine-triggered seizures

* The additional code specifies the type of seizure.

1.2 Taking the headache history

A thorough history is important for any diagnosis, but is particularly important in headache disorders. If the history is taken carefully and skilfully, it is rare for the physical and neurological examinations to alter the diagnosis significantly.

The temporal pattern must be elucidated immediately. For how long has the patient suffered from the type of headache that now takes him or her to the doctor? If the answer is more than 2 years, then it is definitely a primary headache disorder.

The next question is whether the patient has one or more different kinds of headache. This must be elucidated skilfully, because some patients exaggerate the number of different headaches whereas others believe that all their headaches are of one kind, even if they

Box 1.2 is reproduced with permission from the Headache Classification Subcommittee of the International Headache Society (IHS). The International Classification of Headache Disorders (2nd edition). *Cephalagia*, 2004; **24** (**suppl 1**), 1–160.

are different according to ICHD-2 diagnostic criteria. The reason for the consultation must be made clear. Is it because the usual headache is getting worse, or is it because of a new kind of headache? The following information must be obtained about each of the different headaches of the patient. Is it attack-wise or is it more continuous? If attack-wise, does it fulfil criteria for migraine, episodic tension-type headache, cluster headache, trigeminal neuralgia, or other attack-wise headaches? If it is more or less continuous, does it fulfil criteria for chronic tension-type headache, new daily persistent headache, chronic post-traumatic headache, or, most importantly, does the patient have medication overuse? This is defined as taking triptans, ergots, or opioids on more than 9 days per month, or plain analgesics and non-steroidal anti-inflammatory drugs on more than 14 days per month. Does the patient have symptoms other than headache, such as personality change, forgetfulness, speech difficulty, or any symptoms from the extremities that would warn against a secondary cause of the headache?

To classify primary headaches, the following questions are crucial: frequency and duration of attacks, headache severity, is the pain on one or both sides? Is it aggravated by physical activity? The presence of trigger zones and lancinating quality suggest a neuralgia. Is a migraine aura present? And, very importantly, are there accompanying symptoms such as nausea, hypersensitivity to light and sound, or autonomic symptoms such as tearing, stuffed nose, sweating, ptosis, or miosis?

As discussed in Chapter 2 the use of headache diaries, calendars, and other instruments is very useful for an even more precise diagnosis and as a basis for headache management.

1.3 **Examining the headache patient**

It is relatively rare that the examination of headache patients reveals abnormalities. Some doctors drop the examination altogether if the history does not suggest a secondary cause of the headache. However, this is not advisable and may be considered malpractice for several reasons. First of all, it may be extremely serious if a secondary cause such as a brain tumour or arterial hypertension is overlooked. Secondly, patients expect an examination even if their headache history is several years' long. The examination increases considerably the confidence of the patient in the physician and thereby enhances compliance with subsequent treatments. Palpation of the temporal arteries can reveal temporal arteritis, and palpation of the extra-cranial and neck muscles serves to reveal the source of pain in patients with tension-type headache. Ophthalmoscopy can reveal papilloedema, which, in patients with posterior fossa tumours, may be the only neurological abnormality. Mental state examination may reveal dementia, depression, or anxiety, often associated with headache. Blood pressure measurement is indispensable.

1.4 The burden and cost of headache disorders

The World Health Organization (WHO) has published a huge study of the global burden of all diseases. WHO calculates the number of years lost due to premature death, which of course is close to zero for headache disorders. Additionally, WHO calculates the number of years lost due to disability, but only for migraine in the absence of data for other headaches. In terms of disability, migraine is among the top 20 diseases in the world, and for women it is number 12 (Table 1.1). In addition, on the composite measure, disability-adjusted life years (DALY), which is the sum of the years lost due to early death and years lost due to disability, migraine scores highly, especially among females. Women have a twofold greater prevalence of migraine than men, and also experience more frequent and more severe attacks. Therefore, migraine is primarily a female disorder.

Recently the cost of migraine in Europe was calculated in real economic terms as part of a study of brain disorders in Europe. This study included psychiatric as well as neurological diseases and it recorded both the direct health care costs and indirect health costs, such as those due to lost work time. The cost of migraine was 27 000 million euros per year in the EU plus Norway, Switzerland, and Iceland, with a total population of approximately 450 million people. This placed migraine as the number 2 neurological disorder in terms of cost, second only to dementia. The cost of migraine was twice as high as the cost of epilepsy, Parkinson's disease, or multiple sclerosis.

The data on non-migraine headaches were considered too scarce to allow a precise estimate. However, the cost of these headaches was considered to be equal to or larger than the cost of migraine. If this assumption is correct, headache disorders would be as costly as dementia, more costly than stroke and at least three times more costly than any other neurological disease.

These figures may be difficult to grasp, but they illustrate that headache disorders are extremely prevalent and very burdensome to most of the individuals affected. Consequently, they tell the practicing physician to take headache disorders seriously and to treat them with the best available means. New treatments, such as the triptans, need save only very few working days in order to be good business for society. This is without regard to the human suffering that is caused by the severe pain of migraine and other headaches, a factor that should be seen as much more important than the societal cost of these disorders. In this light, it is surprising and disappointing that headache patients remain poorly diagnosed and treated in most countries.

Table 1.1 Years of life lived with a disability (YDLs): Both sexes

Both sexes, all ages	**Rank % of total YDLs**	**Females, all ages**	**Rank % of total YDLs**
1. Unipolar depressive disorders	11.9	1. Unipolar depressive disorders	14.0
2. Hearing loss, adult onset	4.6	2. Iron-deficiency anemia	4.9
3. Iron-deficiency anemia	4.5	3. Hearing loss, adult onset	4.2
4. Chronic obstructive pulmonary disease	3.3	4. Osteoarthritis	3.5
5. Alcohol-use disorders	3.1	5. Chronic obstructive pulmonary disease	2.9
6. Osteoarthritis	3.0	6. Schizophrenia	2.7
7. Schizophrenia	2.8	7. Bipolar affective disorder	2.4
8. Falls	2.8	8. Falls	2.3
9. Bipolar affective disorder	2.5	9. Alzheimer's and other dementias	2.2
10. Asthma	2.1	10. Obstructed labor	2.1
11. Congenital abnormalities	2.1	11. Cataracts	2.0
12. Perinatal conditions	2.0	**12. Migraine**	**2.0**
13. Alzheimer's and other dementias	2.0	13. Congenital abnormalities	1.9
14. Cataracts	1.9	14. Asthma	1.8
15. Road traffic accidents	1.8	15. Perinatal conditions	1.8
16. Protein-energy malnutrition	1.7	16. Chlamydia infection	1.8
17. Cerebrovascular disease	1.7	17. Cerebrovascular disease	1.8
18. HIV/AIDS	1.5	18. Protein-energy malnutrition	1.6
19. Migraine	**1.4**	19. Abortion	1.6
20. Diabetes mellitus	1.4	20. Panic disorder	1.6

Annual WHO report 2001: Mental health: New understanding, New hope % of total YLDs caused by a disorder

Table 1.2 Taking a diagnostic history

Questions to ask in the history	
How many different headaches types do you have? A separate history is needed for each.	
Time questions	• Why consulting now? • How recent in onset? • How frequent, and what temporal pattern (episodic or daily and/or unremitting)? • How long lasting?
Character questions	• Intensity of pain? • Nature and quality of pain? • Site and spread of pain? • Associated symptoms?
Cause questions	• Predisposing and/or trigger factors? • Aggravating and/or relieving factors? • Family history of similar headache?
Response questions	• What does the patient do during the headache? • How much is activity (function) limited or prevented? • What medication has been and is used, in what manner and with what effect?
State of health between attacks	• Completely well, or residual or persisting symptoms? • Concerns, anxieties, fears about recurrent attacks, and/or their cause?
Ref: Steiner TJ, MacGregor EA, Davies PTG (2007). Guidelines for all healthcare professional in the diagnosis and management of migraine, tension-type, cluster and medication overuse headache (3rd edition).	

1.5 Headache research

Thirty years ago little was understood about the neurobiological mechanisms of headache, but over the last three decades headache research has progressed tremendously. We now know that the migraine aura is caused by a cortical spreading depression, that mutation in certain genes can cause migraine via imbalance of ions across the neuronal cell membrane, that messenger molecules such as serotonin (5-hydroxytryptamine, 5HT), nitric oxide (NO), and calcitonin gene-related peptide (CGRP) are strongly involved in migraine mechanisms. The neurobiology of the afferent sensory system responsible for headache is now much better understood, including the role of sensitization of the central pain processing pathways.

All of this progress has been provided by a small number of dedicated research groups and at very small economic cost. In fact, it was recently shown that there is a severe underinvestment in headache research despite the fact that the above-mentioned advances suggest that headache research may be one of the most profitable areas of research investment. There is now a strong movement to persuade the National Institutes of Health in the USA to create a special section for headache in order to stimulate American headache research. The European Commission in Brussels has already acknowledged headache as an important public health problem, in line with recent extensive studies by the WHO. If these new developments are carried on, we can expect major advances in our understanding of the mechanisms of migraine and other headaches, and in our treatment possibilities in the future.

Key references

Andlin-Sobocki P, Jonsson B, Wittchen HU and Olesen J (2005). Cost of disorders of the brain in Europe. *Eur J Neurol* **12 (suppl 1)**, 1–27.

Headache Classification Subcommittee of the International Headache Society (2004). The International Classification of Headache Disorders (2nd edition). *Cephalalgia*, **24 (suppl 1)**, 1–160.

Olesen J (2006). *The Headaches*, 3rd edn. Lippincott Williams & Wilkins, Philadelphia.

Olesen J and Steiner TJ (2004). The International Classification of Headache Disorders, 2nd edn (ICDH-II). *J Neurol Neurosurg Psychiatry* **75**, 808–811.

Sobocki P, Lekander I, Berwick S, Olesen J and Jonsson B (2006). Resource allocation to brain research in Europe (RABRE). *Eur J Neurosci* **24**, 2691–3.

Steiner TJ (2004). Lifting the burden: the global campaign against headache. *Lancet Neurol* **3**, 204–5.

Part 1

Diagnosis

Chapter 2

Migraine

Anne MacGregor

Key points

- Migraine is the commonest cause of severe episodic recurrent headache.
- The diagnosis is based on a history of typical symptoms in the absence of physical signs.
- No tests or investigations can confirm the diagnosis of migraine and their only indication is to exclude secondary headaches.
- Diary cards are an invaluable aid to diagnosis.

2.1 What is migraine?

Migraine is the commonest cause of severe episodic recurrent headache. Attacks typically last between 4 and 72 hours and can occur, on average, every 4–6 weeks. Although migraine is a benign condition, the severity and frequency of attacks can result in significant disability and reduced quality of life, even between attacks.

Typical characteristics of the headache are unilateral location, pulsating quality, moderate or severe intensity, aggravation by routine physical activity, and association with nausea and/or photophobia and phonophobia.

Clinically, an attack of migraine can further be divided into five distinct phases (Figure 2.1):

- Premonitory phase
- Aura
- Headache and associated symptoms
- Resolution
- Recovery/postdromal phase.

Figure 2.1 Migraine: theories of pathogenesis

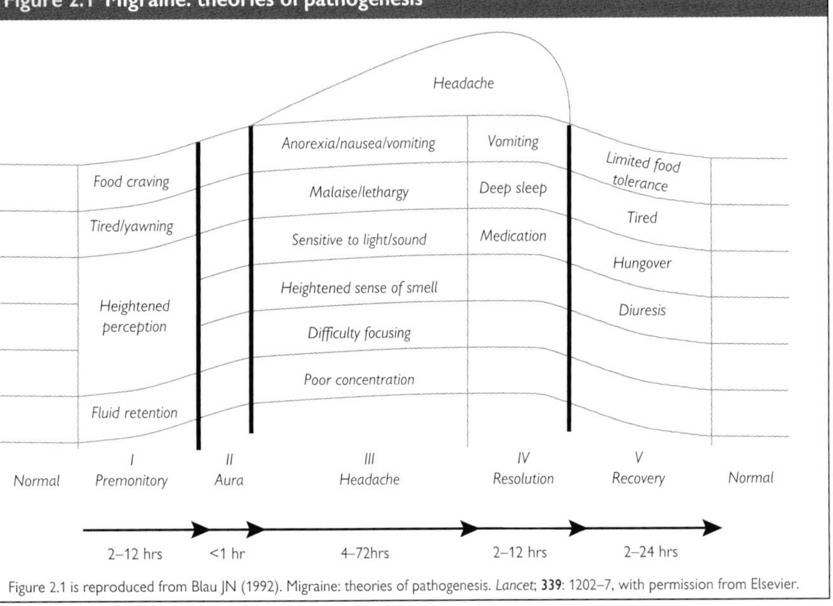

Figure 2.1 is reproduced from Blau JN (1992). Migraine: theories of pathogenesis. *Lancet*; **339**: 1202–7, with permission from Elsevier.

2.1.1 **Premonitory phase**

Not all migraineurs are aware of premonitory symptoms, which can precede attacks of both migraine with and without aura by 12–24 hours. Symptoms are suggestive of hypothalamic disturbance and are distinct from, and unrelated to, the aura. They may include:

- irritability
- feeling 'high' or 'low'
- extreme fatigue and yawning
- dysphasia
- constipation
- hunger and craving for sweets or specific foods
- urinary frequency, thirst, or fluid retention
- neck stiffness
- photophobia and/or phonophobia
- nausea
- difficulty with concentration.

Some premonitory symptoms are incorrectly blamed as triggers for the attack. For example, craving for sweet foods may result in a desire to eat chocolate. A few people feel 'on top of the world' before an attack and rush around, later thinking that the attack was caused by overactivity. In fact, these are signs that the attack has already begun. Recognition of these premonitory symptoms can be of enormous benefit, because avoiding known trigger factors during this time may be all that is necessary to stop the attack from developing further.

2.1.2 **Aura**

Symptoms of aura gradually develop over 5–20 minutes, last for less than 1 hour, and usually resolve completely before the onset of headache. Atypical or permanent symptoms warrant further investigation.

Visual symptoms

Homonymous visual symptoms are most common, experienced in 99% of auras. Aura without visual symptoms is rare. Visual symptoms are usually symmetrical, affecting one hemifield of both eyes, although subjectively they may appear to affect only one eye. The typical 'fortification spectra' begins with a bright migrainous scotoma,starting as a small spot and gradually increasing in size to assume a C shape (Figure 2.2). It often develops scintillating edges that appear as zigzags or fortifications—a term coined in the late eighteenth century because the visual disturbances resembled a fortified town surrounded by bastions. Visual symptoms can begin either in the centre or in the periphery of the visual field, gradually spreading across the field of vision and increasing in size over a period of 5–30 minutes, and resolve within 60 minutes.

Figure 2.2

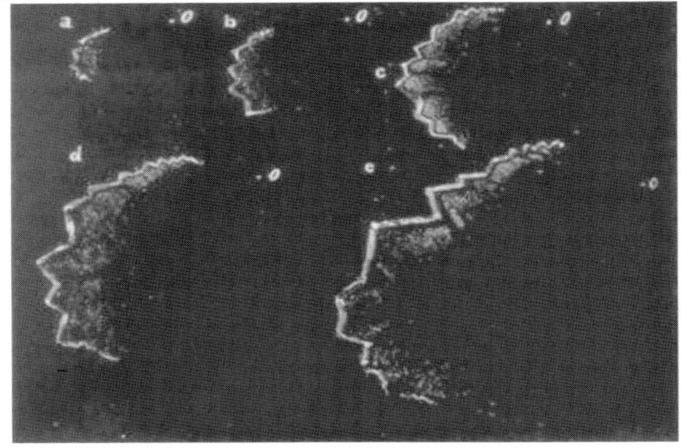

Figure 2.2 is reproduced from Airy H (1870). On a distinct form of transient hemiopsia. *Phil Trans Roy Soc*; **160**: 247–64.

Sensory symptoms

Sensory disturbance occurs in around one-third of auras and is usually associated with visual symptoms. The symptoms are typically positive, for instance a tingling sensation of 'pins and needles'. Migraine symptoms have a characteristic unilateral distribution affecting one arm, slowly spreading over 5 minutes, or more proximally from the hand to affect the mouth and tongue (i.e. cheiro-oral distribution). The leg is rarely affected in migraine. Motor weakness is not a feature of typical migraine with aura.

Other symptoms

Speech disturbance and motor symptoms can also be present (18% and 6% respectively), but only in association with visual and/or sensory symptoms. Symptoms usually follow one another in succession, beginning with visual, followed by sensory symptoms, dysphasia, and weakness. Each symptom lasts from 5 to 60 minutes.

2.1.3 **Headache and associated symptoms**

The throbbing headache is typically unilateral, sometimes changing sides during an attack, but may be bilateral. It is aggravated by movement of the head and accompanied by nausea or vomiting, photophobia and/or phonophobia. Although some sufferers can continue limited activities, many have to retire to bed in a darkened room until symptoms subside.

2.1.4 **Resolution**

Other than with effective medication, the natural course of migraine is to resolve with sleep. Some attacks, particularly in children, improve after vomiting.

2.1.5 **Recovery/postdromal phase**

After the headache has gone, most migraineurs feel drained and washed out for a further day. Rarely, they feel very energetic and even euphoric.

2.2 **Epidemiology**

2.2.1 **Prevalence and incidence**

Globally, the lifetime prevalence of migraine is around 8% in men and 25% in women, and only minor variation has been reported among races.

The incidence of migraine is equal in both sexes before puberty. At puberty, the incidence of migraine without aura rises in females, with 10–20% of women with migraine reporting their first attack during the year of menarche. This sex difference becomes greater with increasing age, peaking during the early forties and declining thereafter.

2.2.2 **Age at onset**

The first attack of migraine usually occurs during the teens and early twenties, with 90% of attacks occurring before age 40.

2.2.3 **Type of migraine**

- About 70–80% of migraineurs experience attacks of migraine *without* aura (formerly known as common or simple migraine)
- 10% have migraine *with* aura (formerly known as classical or focal migraine)
- 15–20% have both types of attack
- Less than 1% of attacks are of aura alone, with no ensuing headache.

Patients may, at different times, have attacks of migraine with aura and migraine without aura. They may, over a lifetime, change from a predominance of one subtype to the other. In contrast to migraine without aura, which is most prevalent during a woman's reproductive years and improves in later life, the prevalence of migraine with aura increases with age, accompanying around 13% of attacks in the age group of 18–29 years, increasing up to 41% of attacks in people with migraine aged 70 years or above.

2.2.4 **Frequency of attacks**

Migraine is a fluctuating condition. A longitudinal study of 73 migraineurs over 40 years showed that attack frequency was variable with time, sometimes with long episodes of remission. A 12-year epidemiological follow-up study demonstrated remission in 42%, decreased frequency in 38%, and increased frequency in only 20%.

2.3 Diagnosing migraine

Diagnostic criteria for migraine with and without aura are shown in Boxes 2.1 and 2.2. However, these criteria are better designed for clinical trials rather than clinical practice, as they do not take account of the patterns of occurrence of attacks.

2.3.1 History

Headaches are not mutually exclusive, so a useful opening question is 'How many different headaches do you have?'. Take a separate history for each headache.

Migraine can be screened using five predictors:

- pulsating headache
- duration 4–72 hours
- unilateral
- associated nausea
- disability.

If three predictors are present, the likelihood ratio for migraine is 3.5 (95% confidence interval [CI] 1.3–9.2), increasing to 24 (95% CI 1.5–388) if four predictors are present.

Box 2.1 International Headache Society diagnostic criteria: migraine without aura

A. At least five attacks fulfilling criteria B–D

B. Headache attacks lasting 4–72 hours (untreated or treated unsuccessfully)*

C. Headache has at least two of the following characteristics:

1. unilateral location*
2. pulsating quality
3. moderate or severe pain intensity
4. aggravation by or causing avoidance of routine physical activity (e.g. walking or climbing stairs)

D. During headache at least one of the following:

1. nausea and/or vomiting*
2. photophobia and phonophobia

E. Not attributed to another disorder

(history and examination do not suggest a secondary headache disorder or, if they do, it is ruled out by appropriate investigations, or headache attacks do not occur for the first time in close temporal relation to the other disorder)

* **In children**, attacks may be shorter-lasting, headache is more commonly bilateral, and gastrointestinal disturbance is more prominent.

Box 2.2 International Headache Society diagnostic criteria: migraine with aura

A. At least two attacks fulfilling criteria B–D

B. Aura consisting of at least one of the following, but no motor weakness:
   1. fully reversible visual symptoms including positive features (e.g. flickering lights, spots, or lines) and/or negative features (i.e. loss of vision)
   2. fully reversible sensory symptoms including positive features (i.e. pins and needles) and/or negative features (i.e. numbness)
   3. fully reversible dysphasic speech disturbance

C. At least two of the following:
   1. homonymous visual symptoms and/or unilateral sensory symptoms
   2. at least one aura symptom develops gradually over ≥5 minutes and/or different aura symptoms occur in succession over ≥5 minutes
   3. each symptom lasts ≥5 and ≤60 minutes

D. Headache fulfilling criteria B–D for migraine without aura (see Box 2.1) begins during the aura or follows aura within 60 minutes

E. Not attributed to another disorder

If the screening questions suggest migraine, typical responses to the following questions can confirm the diagnosis:

- 'How old were you when you had your first attack?' Migraine starts in the young; it is unusual for a first attack to occur in a patient aged over 55 years. However, the older patient may seek help for exacerbation of migraine after several years of respite.
- 'How often do you have an attack?' Migraine is an episodic condition. If the patient complains of daily or near daily headaches, then the diagnosis of the primary headache is unlikely to be migraine. However, patients may have had attacks of migraine for many years which they have controlled, but daily headaches are the reason why they have sought help, particularly if the superimposed migraine attacks have also become more frequent and less responsive to treatment.
- 'How long does the attack last?' Most attacks last for part of a day, but some may last up to 3 days.
- 'How do you feel when you haven't got a headache?' Most patients answer 'Fine'. If the patient has symptoms between attacks, look for additional headaches or other pathology.

- 'Describe a typical attack?' Most patients with migraine describe a one-sided throbbing headache with nausea and/or vomiting, photophobia, and phonophobia, which may be preceded by prodromal symptoms and/or aura.
- 'What do you do when you have an attack?' Some migraineurs manage to struggle through the day and collapse in bed when they get home. Others cannot get to work or have to leave work early. They typically retire to bed in a quiet, darkened room and try to lie still as movement can aggravate pain and nausea.
- 'What do the headaches stop you doing?' Frequent attacks can result in severe disability during an attack as well as through fear of an impending attack. Such situations warrant more aggressive management than mild, infrequent migraine.

Diagnosing migraine aura

Premonitory symptoms are often misdiagnosed as migraine aura, because both are 'warnings' of imminent headache. Premonitory symptoms tend to be vague, preceding the headache by several hours and often continuing for the duration of the attack. Visual symptoms such as generalized 'spots before the eyes', 'flashing lights', or blurring of vision often occur during both the premonitory and headache phases. In contrast, aura is distinct—when asked to describe their aura, patients typically draw a zigzag line in the air, representing the scintillations.

Aura can be identified by a positive response to the question: 'Have you ever had visual disturbances lasting 5–60 minutes followed by headache?'.

Contemporaneous recording of symptoms is recommended, as common mistakes that patients make when describing aura include reports of sudden onset when it is gradual, of monocular disturbances that are homonymous, describing sensory loss as weakness, and incorrect duration.

2.3.2 **Examination**

A diagnosis of migraine is usually clear from the patient's history, but the examination is necessary to ensure that there is no major brain pathology. A brief but thorough physical and a neurological examination is essential, with particular emphasis placed on the relevant systems. Careful fundoscopic examination for papilloedema or other abnormalities is especially useful to evaluate for secondary headaches. Blood pressure should also be measured as, although hypertension is rarely a cause of headache, most patients think it is.

2.3.3 **Investigations**

If patients meet the criteria for a primary headache disorder and have a normal neurological examination, further diagnostic testing generally is not helpful. Many people expect to have their migraine investigated with a brain scan. Since no abnormalities have been identified on neurological examination or other investigations in typical migraine, there is no place for investigations other than those indicated to exclude suspected secondary headache resulting from underlying pathology.

Imaging should be considered for cases of undefined headache, atypical symptoms, persistent neurological or psychopathological abnormalities, or abnormal findings on neurological examination. Prolonged aura, especially aura persisting after resolution of the headache, and aura involving motor weakness, should be investigated. Amongst these cases are a very small number of families expressing recognized genes for familial hemiplegic migraine.

2.4 Aids to diagnosis

Many specialists advocate the use of a symptom diary, which patients can use at home to establish a temporal pattern for their headache. A record of migraine will show attacks occurring episodically with days in between when the patient is headache free (Figure 2.3). Symptoms of non-migraine headache may also be apparent. A pattern of attacks may be obvious (days of the week, time of day), revealing potential triggers (sleeping late at weekends, missed meals, etc.). Use of acute drugs can be checked for optimal dosing. Frequent use (10 days or more per month) of acute medication is an alert for medication overuse headache.

Figure 2.3 Example of a monthly migraine diary

Date	Day	Headache or Migraine	Severity	Time Started	Nausea	Vomiting	What treatment did you take	Time taken
1	MON							
2	TUE							
3	WED							
4	THU							
5	FRI	headache	mild	1 pm	No	No	Nothing	
6	SAT	migraine	severe	4 am	Yes	No	Triptan	4 am & 1pm
7	SUN	migraine	moderate	7 am	Yes	No	Triptan	7 am
8	MON							
9	TUE	headache	moderate	10 am	No	No	Analgesic	10 am
10	WED							
11	THU							
12	FRI							
13	SAT							
14	SUN							
15	MON							

Key references

Detsky ME, McDonald DR, Baerlocker MO, Tomlinson GA, McCory DC and Booth CM (2006). Does this patient with headache have a migraine or need neuroimaging? *JAMA* **296**,1274–83.

Gervil M, Ulrich V, Olesen J and Russell M (1998). Screening for migraine in the general population: validation of a simple questionnaire. *Cephalalgia* **18**, 342–8.

Headache Classification Subcommittee of the International Headache Society (2004). The International Classification of Headache Disorders (2nd edition). *Cephalalgia* **24(suppl 1)**, 1–160.

Lyngberg AC, Rasmussen BK, Jorgensen T and Jensen R (2005). Prognosis of migraine and tension-type headache: a population-based follow-up study. *Neurology* **65**, 580–5.

Steiner TJ, MacGregor EA and Davies PTG (2007). Guidelines for all healthcare professional in the diagnosis and management of migraine, tension-type, cluster and medication overuse headache (3rd edn). Available at: http://www.bash.org.uk [accessed 11 Nov 2007].

Stovner L, Hagen K, Jensen R, Katsarava Z, Lipton R, Scher A *et al.* (2007). The global burden of headache: a documentation of headache prevalence and disability worldwide. *Cephalalgia* **27**, 193–210.

Chapter 3

Tension-type headache

Rigmor Jensen

Key points

- Tension-type headache is the most frequent primary headache and equals migraine in terms of cost.
- Tension-type headache is subdivided into three groups according to frequency.
- Tension-type headache is usually a bilateral, pressing, mild to moderate headache without specific features.
- The most frequent differential diagnosis is migraine without aura and medication overuse headache.
- A detailed history and examination is mandatory.
- A symptom diary kept for at least 4 weeks is a useful aid to diagnosis.

3.1 Introduction

Tension-type headache (TTH) is a primary headache and is now subdivided into three groups: an infrequent form occurring for less than 12 days per year, a frequent episodic form lasting for between 12 and 179 days per year, and a chronic form lasting for 180 days per year or more. Epidemiological studies have revealed that, in total, the infrequent form is the most prevalent headache, but it should probably be regarded more as a nuisance than as a disease.

TTH is characterized by a mild to moderate headache that is not associated with the typical debilitating migraine symptoms of nausea, vomiting, photophobia, and phonophobia (International Classification of Headache Disorders, 2nd edition [ICHD-II]) (Box 3.1). Most patients describe their tension-type headache as their normal milder headaches in contrast to their major headaches, migraine or cluster headaches, for which they usually seek medical assistance.

Patients with TTH seek less medical help than migraineurs. In a population study, only 16% of patients with tension-type headache had been in contact with their general practitioner because of the headache, compared with 56% of migraineurs. When data are corrected for the much higher prevalence of TTH, the total use of medical contacts is

Box 3.1 Diagnostic criteria for frequent episodic tension-type headache (IHCD-II)

A. At least 10 episodes occurring on ≥1 but <15 days per month for at least 3 months (≥12 and <180 days per year) and fulfilling criteria B–D
B. Headache lasting from 30 min to 7 days
C. Headache has at least two of the following characteristics:
   1. Bilateral location
   2. Pressing/tightening (non-pulsating) quality
   3. Mild or moderate intensity
   4. Not aggravated by routine physical activity such as walking or climbing stairs
D. Both of the following:
   1. No nausea or vomiting (anorexia may occur)
   2. No more than one of photophobia or phonophobia
E. Not attributed to another disorder

54% higher for tension-type headache than for migraine. Severely affected patients with TTH usually see numerous doctors and spend large sums of money on so-called alternative treatments, living for decades without effective pain relief.

3.2 Epidemiology

TTH varies considerably in frequency, duration, and severity, from rare shortlasting episodes of discomfort to frequent, longlasting, or even continuous disabling headaches. Unlike migraine, there is a clear and positive correlation between the frequency and severity of TTH. In its infrequent mild form, TTH may be a nuisance, but is not regarded as a disease by the affected persons or their doctors. In its frequent and severe forms, it becomes distressing and socially disturbing owing to the constant pain, surpassing the effects of migraine and cluster headache. Considering all patients with TTH as a homogeneous group may be misleading.

The lifetime prevalence of TTH was as high as 78% in a population-based study in Denmark, but the vast majority (59%) had infrequent episodic TTH (less than one headache day per month) and were not in need of medical care. Some 24–37% of the population have TTH once a month or more, 10% have it weekly, and 2–3% have chronic TTH, usually for the greater part of their lifetime.

The male:female ratio of TTH is 4:5, indicating that, unlike migraine, females are only slightly more affected than men. In both sexes the prevalence seems to peak between 30 and 39 years of age, and appears to decrease with advancing years.

The average age of onset of TTH is higher than in migraine, namely 25–30 years in cross-sectional epidemiological studies. TTH, like other chronic headaches, is probably a lifelong disorder as prevalence tends to increase until the fifth decade, with only a minor decline with increasing age.

The prognosis of patients with TTH is fairly positive. In a recent 12-year follow-up study of a general population, Lyngberg *et al.* (2005a) found that 47% of subjects with chronic TTH had remission, whereas 12% with episodic TTH developed the chronic form. Poor outcome was associated with baseline chronic TTH, coexisting migraine, not being married, and sleeping problems.

3.3 **Diagnosis**

TTH is a fairly featureless headache and may mimic other primary or secondary headaches. Patients with pure episodic TTH rarely attend headache centres; only 16% of TTH sufferers in the general population seek medical help for TTH, and only 3% seek specialized care.

Case definitions in TTH may also be difficult because the condition may overlap with mild attacks of migraine. Some patients and doctors have difficulty distinguishing between different types of attack, and in clinical populations patients may have up to five different ICHD-II diagnoses. A detailed interview, a clinical neurological examination, and use of a diagnostic diary for several weeks are therefore important. The questions in Table 1.2 are very important to facilitate the diagnostic process.

In the general population, 94% of migraineurs also experience TTH, and 56% experience frequent episodic TTH. In contrast, TTH occurs with similar prevalence in those with and without migraine, leading to the assumption that migraine may trigger TTH, whereas TTH may not trigger migraine. This co-morbidity may explain why there has been so much controversy about TTH as a clinical entity and why the existence of TTH has been questioned.

3.4 **History**

Patients with TTH usually describe their pain as a 'dull', 'non-pulsating' headache. The pain is typically bilateral (90%) and a strict unilateral location calls for increased attention, and secondary causative factors for headache should be considered. The pain quality is pressing and tightening, and terms such as a sensation of 'tightness', 'pressure', or 'soreness' are used. The pain is often described as an external pain coming from the outside, and some patients refer to a 'band' or 'cap' compressing their head, whereas others mention a heavy 'weight' over their head and/or their shoulders.

Figure 3.1 Diagnostic diary from a patient with TTH and coexisting migraine

After each question put one x in the box which is most appropriate.

Name: Mrs. HANSEN Birthday: Nov 10.1962

2007	Date:	12/1	13/1	15/1	16/1	24/1	1/2	6/2
When did the headache begin?	Indicate nearest hour:	7	7	10	7	14	10	7
Just before the headache began, was there any disturbance of	Vision:							
	other senses:							
Was the headache	rightsided:			X	X			
	leftsided:							
	both sides:	X	X			X	X	X
Was the headache	pulsating/throbbing:			X	X			
	pressing/tightening:	X	X			X	X	X
Was the headache * See below	mild:	X				X	X	
	moderate:		X					X
	severe:			X				
Did the headache change with physical activity such as walking stairs	worse:			X				
	unchanged:	X			X	X	X	X
	better:		X					
Did you suffer from nausea?	no:	X	X			X	X	X
	mild:				X			
	moderate:			X				
	severe:							
Were you bothered by light?	no:	X	X			X	X	X
	mildly:				X			
	moderately:			X				
	severely:							
Were you bothered by sounds?	no:	X	X		X	X	X	X
	mildly:			X				
	moderately:							
	severely:							
When did the headache disappear?	Indicate nearest hour:	22	20	22	10	20	21	17
Did anything provoke this attack?	specify:							
Did you take any medicine? Mention each different compound, how much you took, and when you took it (nearest hour).	name:							
	how much:							
	time:							
	name:							
	how much:							
	time:							

* **Mild: Does** not inhibit work performance or other activities
Moderate: Inhibits, but does not prohibit work perfomance and other activities
Severe: Prohibits work and other activities

In one study, TTH was of a pressing quality in 78% of patients, mild or moderate in 99%, bilateral in 90%, and 72% had no aggravation with physical activity. The accompanying symptoms of nausea, photophobia, and phonophobia occur only rarely and, if present, are usually mild. The presence of nausea may again raise suspicion of migraine or medication overuse. In addition, nausea and aggravation by physical activity are important predictors of a migraine attack. Patients suffering from both conditions can learn to discriminate between TTH and migraine by these accompanying symptoms.

For diagnosis the use of diaries for at least 4 weeks is highly recommended. As described in Chapter 2 (see Figure 2.3), a detailed diagnostic diary is useful initially with a simplified calendar for the

Figure 3.1 adapted from Russell M, Rasmussen BK, Brennum J, Iversen H, Jensen R, Olesen J, (1992). Presentation of a new instrument. The diagnostic headache diary. *Cephalagia* **12**, 369–374, with permission from Blackwell Publishing.

follow-up subsequent to the diagnosis. An example of diagnostic diary for a patient suffering from frequent episodic TTH and coexisting migraine without aura is illustrated in Figure 3.1. Detailed studies of the diagnostic and educational values of such diaries are in progress in Europe and could pave the way for further systematic studies between different clinics and countries.

A detailed history of any possible triggers is also of utmost importance, especially in the episodic subforms. As in migraine, elimination of any possible triggers, such as dental pathology, a cyclical hormonal relationship, sinus disease, unphysiological working conditions, posture, unbalanced meals, and inadequate sleep, can reduce the frequency of attacks but, in practice, are difficult to identify.

In summary, a secondary headache should always be considered in all patients consulting for headache; most frequently medication overuse headache but also serious life-threatening cases may mimic TTH. The major differential diagnoses are listed in Table 3.1.

Table 3.1 Warning symptoms, possible differential diagnosis to the primary headaches, and suggested strategy (any new headache in an individual patient should be treated with caution)

Warning feature	Differential diagnosis	Suggested investigation
Thunderclap: abrupt onset of a new headache	Subarachnoid haemorrhage	CT-C and MRA, and, if negative, a lumbar puncture
Atypical aura (>1 h or motor symptoms)	Migraine, TIA, or stroke	Detailed history, CT-C or MRI
New headache in a patient older than 40 years	Intracranial tumour or temporal arteritis	Detailed history, CT-C or MRI as well as blood tests
New headache in a pre-pubertal child	Intracranial tumour	Detailed history, and eventually MRI
Nausea and progressive headache frequency	Medication overuse headache	Detailed medication registration and a new neurological examination
Intense headache aggravated by physical activity and accompanying symptoms	Migraine	Detailed history and diagnostic diary
Progressive headache accompanied by focal neurological or cognitive symptoms or signs	Intracranial space-occupying lesion	Detailed examination and CT-C or MRI
Progressive pulsating headache, tinnitus, and transient visual disturbances	Idiopathic intracranial hypertension	MRA and MRV, and, if normal, a lumbar puncture and opening pressure

CT-C, computed tomography of the cerebrum; MRA, magnetic resonance angiography; MRI, magnetic resonance imaging; MRV, magnetic resonance venography; TIA, transient ischaemic attack.

3.5 Examination

Although diagnostic tests are widely used in patients with TTH , they are seldom indicated unless atypical features such as marked treatment resistance are present. In addition to the primary diagnosis, a careful history is also important to uncover coexisting diseases such as depression or anxiety. In tension-type headache, the general examination should also include manual palpation of the pericranial muscles, particularly the temporal, masseteric, neck and sternoclei domastoid muscles. One or two fingers should be used, with moderate to firm pressure and small rotating movements. Pain can be scored on a scale of 0–3 based on verbal response and observation of the patient (Figure 3.2). This will demonstrate any peripheral muscular factor to the patient, and indicates the potential benefit of physical training and relaxation therapy.

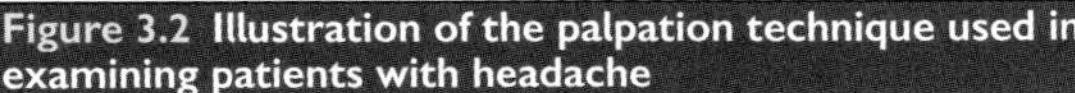

Figure 3.2 Illustration of the palpation technique used in examining patients with headache

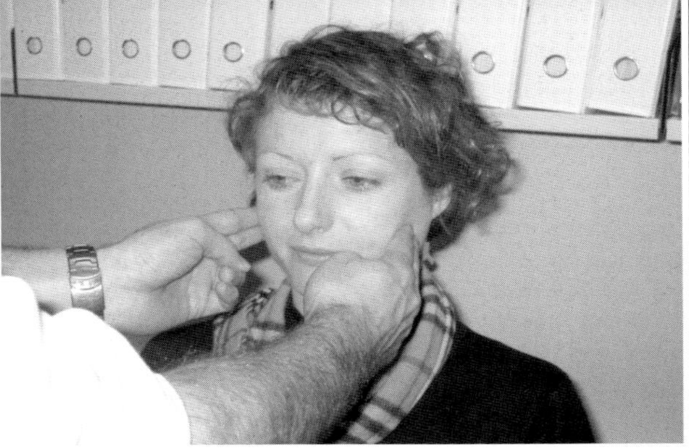

Use second and third finger, and use and exert mild pressure and small rotating movements. Generally use bilateral palpation. For palpation of neck insertions, you need one hand to support the head and one to do the palpation under the cranium. The muscles that are usually examined are the temporal mesenteric and trapezius muscles plus neck insertions. The whole examination takes only about 2 min, and it is very effective in demonstrating the possible source of pain in tension-type headache.

3.6 Investigations

In patients with recent changes in headache pattern, abnormal neurological findings, weight loss or marked weight increase, personality, or cognitive changes, blood samples and neuroimaging with computed tomography or magnetic resonance imaging should be undertaken. Neuroimaging of the cervical and/or lumbar spine is not usually recommended as the specificity in relation to headache is poor and often misleading.

As indicated in Chapter 2, a complete general and neurological examination, including blood pressure, cardiac auscultation, body weight, inspection of the lumbar and cervical spine and fundi, is essential in all newly referred patients with headache. Only very rarely are abnormalities leading to a secondary cause of the headache identified, but it is mandatory to remain aware of symptoms and signs of sinister headaches, and also to let patients know that they have been seriously considered and examined by their doctor.

3.7 Conclusion

An accurate diagnosis, in which the individual headache episode is distinguished from migraine and from a secondary headache, especially medication overuse, is essential. The use of a diagnostic headache diary is mandatory before treatment planning, and the prevention of headache consists of the elimination of possible triggers. Analysis of psychological triggers or co-morbidity with depressive disorders is also mandatory before treatment is initiated.

Key references

Bendtsen L and Jensen R (2006). Tension-type headache: the most common, but also the most neglected, headache disorder. *Curr Opin Neurol* **19**, 305–9.

Castillio J, Murioz P, Guitera V and Pasqual J (1999). Epidemiology of chronic daily headache in the general population. *Headache* **39**, 190–6.

Goebel H, Petersen-Braun M and Soyka D (1994). The epidemiology of headache in Germany: a nationwide survey of a representative sample on the basis of the headache classification of the International Headache Society. *Cephalalgia* **14**, 97–106.

Headache Classification Committee of the International Headache Society (1988). Classification and diagnostic criteria for headache disorders, cranial neuralgias and facial pain. *Cephalalgia* **8(suppl 7)**, 1–96.

Headache Classification Subcommittee of the International Headache Society (2004). The international classification of headache disorders, 2nd edition. *Cephalalgia* **24(suppl 1)**, 1–160.

Jensen R (1999). Pathophysiological mechanisms of tension-type headache. A review of epidemiological and experimental studies. *Cephalalgia* **19**, 602–21.

Lyngberg AC, Rasmussen BK, Jørgensen T and Jensen R (2005a). Prognosis of migraine and tension-type headache. A population-based follow-up study. *Neurology* **65**, 580–5.

Lyngberg AC, Rasmussen BK, Jørgensen T and Jensen R (2005b). Incidence of primary headache: a Danish epidemiologic follow-up study. *Am J Epidemiol* **161**, 1066–73.

Rasmussen BK, Jensen R, Schroll M and Olesen J (1991). Epidemiology of headache in a general population—a prevalence study. *J Clin Epidemiol* **44**, 1147–57.

Steiner T, Paemeliere K, Jensen R *et al.* (2007). European principles of management of common headache disorders in primary care. *J Headache Pain* **8**, S3–47.

Tassorelli C, Sances G, Allena M, Ghiotto N, Bendtsen L, Olesen J, Nappi G, Jensen R. (2008). The usefulness and applicability of a basic headache diary before first consultation—results of a pilot study conducted in two centres. *Cephalalgia* (2008).

Chapter 4

Cluster and other trigeminal autonomic cephalalgias

Anna S Cohen

Key points

- Trigeminal autonomic cephalalgias (TACs) are characterized by attacks of severe unilateral pain and accompanying ipsilateral cranial autonomic features.
- Attacks of paroxysmal hemicrania (PH) and SUNCT (short-lasting unilateral neuralgiform headache attacks with conjunctival injection and tearing) are more frequent and shorter than in cluster headache (CH).
- In CH, the episodic form prevails; in other TACs, the chronic form is more common.
- Characteristic triggers for attacks include alcohol for CH, and cutaneous triggers for SUNCT.
- All TACs are generally primary syndromes, but underlying lesions such as pituitary tumours and posterior fossa lesions must be excluded.
- Brain magnetic resonance imaging is the recommended investigation for all new diagnoses of TAC.

4.1 Introduction

Trigeminal autonomic cephalalgias (TACs) are a group of rare primary headache syndromes that include cluster headache (CH), paroxysmal hemicrania (PH), and SUNCT (short-lasting unilateral neuralgiform headache attacks with conjunctival injection and tearing) and SUNA (short-lasting unilateral neuralgiform headache attacks with cranial autonomic symptoms). Although rare, they are important to recognize because of their excellent but highly selective response to treatment. They share the same features in their phenotype of headache attacks, which is a severe unilateral orbital, periorbital, or temporal pain, with associated ipsilateral cranial autonomic symptoms, such as conjunctival injection, lacrimation, nasal blockage, rhinorrhoea, eyelid oedema, and ptosis. The International Headache Society (IHS) has set out diagnostic criteria. The distinction between the syndromes is made on duration and frequency of attacks (Table 4.1). Between SUNCT and SUNA, the distinction is in the presence of cranial autonomic features such as conjunctival injection and tearing. Typical migrainous features such as photophobia and phonophobia are seen, but they are usually unilateral as opposed to the bilateral symptoms of migraine attack. TACs can be episodic or chronic.

4.2 Diagnosis of TACs

The diagnosis of TACs is based primarily on the history. A detailed account of the side, site, and type of pain is elicited, as well as the accompanying autonomic symptoms. The frequency and duration of the attacks may help to distinguish between the TACs, as may specific details such as wakening the patient at night (CH), absolute response to indometacin (PH), and cutaneous triggers (SUNCT).

Although these syndromes are for the most part primary headache disorders, a full past medical history is obtained and a detailed neurological examination is performed in order to rule out an underlying structural brain lesion or cause for a secondary TAC. Cranial imaging such as magnetic resonance imaging (MRI), and blood tests may be useful to identify or rule out any underlying pathology in cases where the attacks are not typical of a particular TAC phenotype, although not all symptomatic TACs have an atypical presentation.

4.3 Cluster Headache (CH)

CH is the commonest of the TACs, with a prevalence of about 0.3%, and male:female ratio of 3.5–7:1. CH typically occurs in adulthood or middle age, but can present in childhood or in the elderly. The incidence diminishes with age.

4.3.1 Phenotype

The attacks of CH are stereotypical, being severe or excruciating, lasting 15–180 min, occurring once every other day up to eight times per day, and associated with ipsilateral autonomic symptoms. The headache is strictly unilateral but it may alternate sides. Most patients are agitated during an attack, in contrast to migraine where movement exacerbates the pain. Most patients report a circadian predictability of the onset of attacks, with 73% reporting nocturnal attacks in one study.

Table 4.1 Clinical feature of TACs				
	CH	PH	SUNCT	SUNA
Sex ratio F:M	1:3.5–7	2.2–2.4:1	1:2	2:1
Type of pain	Stabbing, boring	Throbbing, boring, stabbing	Burning, stabbing, sharp	
Severity	Excruciating	Excruciating	Severe to excruciating	
Site	Orbit, temple	Orbit, temple	Orbital, temporal, periorbital, anywhere on ipsilateral side of head	
Attack frequency	1/alternate day—8/day	1–40/day (>5/day >50% of the time)	3–200/day	
Duration of attack	15–180 min	2–30 min	5–240 s for single stabs, longer for groups of stabs or saw-tooth attacks	
Autonomic features	Yes	Yes	Yes†	Yes†
Migrainous features*	Yes	Yes	Yes, usually associated with migrainous biology	
Agitation during attack	Yes	Yes	Occasional	
Interictal pain	Rarely	Occasional	Yes	
Alcohol trigger	Yes	No	No	
Cutaneous triggers	No	No	Yes	
Indometacin effect	–	++	–	

Ref: Goadsby *et al.* (2007). *Curr Neurol Neurosci Rep* **7**, 117–25.

CH, cluster headache; PH, paroxysmal hemicrania; SUNCT, short-lasting unilateral neuralgiform headache attacks with conjunctival injection and tearing; SUNA, short-lasting unilateral neuralgiform headache attacks with cranial autonomic symptoms.

* Nausea, photophobia or phonophobia.

† Patients with SUNCT have both conjunctival injection and lacrimation; patients with SUNA have either conjunctival injection or lacrimation.

++ indicates absolute response to indometacin.

Cluster headache can be either episodic (ECH), or chronic (CCH). ECH takes the form of bouts or cluster periods, with a period of remission lasting for at least 1 month, and affects the majority of sufferers (85–90%). Bouts are typically around 8 weeks long and occur annually. In CCH, there are attacks for at least 1 year, with remissions no longer than 1 month. During a bout of ECH and in the CCH subtype, attacks may be triggered by alcohol, histamine, or glyceryl trinitrate, usually within an hour in CH.

A family history is possible in CH. There have been case reports and linkage studies of families with CH, and it has been suggested that an autosomal dominant gene has a role in some families. The phenotype of CH may be more atypical in familial disease.

4.3.2 **Examination**

The examination in CH is usually normal. Any abnormal findings on general or neurological examination should alert the clinician to a secondary cause for CH.

4.3.3 **Diagnosis**

Diagnosis is based on IHS criteria for the phenotype of attacks. CH can coexist with migraine in up to 26% of patients, and generally the phenotypes of each syndrome are easily discernible. CH itself may be associated with typically migrainous features such as nausea, vomiting, photophobia, or phonophobia. It can also be associated with an aura, although only 36% of patients with CH and aura had a history of migraine, either with or without aura.

4.3.4 **Secondary/symptomatic CH**

CH is usually a primary headache syndrome. Underlying causes for CH are uncommon and include carotid artery or intracranial arterial dissection, in which case an ipsilateral Horner's syndrome may be mistaken for the autonomic symptoms associated with the CH attack. Other causes of secondary CH include pituitary tumours, pontine lesion in multiple sclerosis, arteriovenous malformations and other space-occupying lesions, and as a post-traumatic phenomenon. It is noted that secondary CH can be either episodic or chronic.

4.3.5 **Investigations**

Although there is biochemical evidence of derangement in serum levels of melatonin, testosterone, cortisol, and thyrotropin, these are not assessed routinely in clinical practice. The exception to this is measuring the prolactin level. This is raised in prolactinoma, which can cause symptomatic CH and other headache syndromes.

MRI of the brain with contrast should be performed in order to rule out a pituitary lesion. In patients with persistent ptosis and suspicion of a Horner's syndrome, the investigations should include imaging of the carotid arteries.

4.4 **Paroxysmal hemicrania (PH)**

PH is less common than CH, with only one case of PH-like syndrome in a study of 1838 people.

4.4.1 **Phenotype**

The attacks are shorter and more frequent than in CH. The pain is reported in the ophthalmic trigeminal distribution, although it can also involve any part of the head. The headache is strictly unilateral, although the attacks can alternate sides. The headache usually lasts for 2–30 min, but can go on for up to 4 h. Interictal discomfort or pain is present in up to 60% of patients. In one study, 27 of 31 patients noted at least one migrainous feature of photophobia, nausea, or vomiting during an attack. Some 85% of a large series were restless or agitated during attacks.

The frequency of attacks in PH is high, ranging from 1 to 40 daily. Two prospective studies have shown frequencies off 11 to 14 daily. The attacks occur regularly throughout the 24-h period, without the nocturnal predominance seen in CH.

Although the majority of attacks are spontaneous, approximately 10% of attacks may be precipitated mechanically, by bending or rotating the head. Attacks may also be provoked by external pressure against the greater occipital nerve. Alcohol triggers headaches in 7% of patients. An association between PH and menstruation has been reported.

About 20% of patients have episodic PH (EPH) with bouts and remissions as in ECH. The remaining 80% have chronic PH (CPH). Notably, in PH the chronic form dominates the clinical presentation, in contrast to CH, in which the episodic form prevails.

PH can coexist with migraine. Although familial PH is rare, it has been reported.

4.4.2 **Examination**

The general and neurological examination in PH is usually normal, as in CH. Any abnormality should alert the clinician to investigate for an underlying cause of secondary PH.

4.4.3 **Diagnosis**

The diagnosis of PH is based on the IHS criteria for the phenotype of attacks, plus an absolute response of the attacks to indometacin. This is ideally administered as the modified *Indotest*; with 100 mg intramuscular indometacin delivered against a blinded saline placebo.

4.4.4 **Secondary/symptomatic PH**

As with CH, PH is generally a primary headache syndrome. However, it has been reported secondary to pituitary lesions, after trauma, after carotid aneurysm embolization, and a PH-like syndrome without autonomic symptoms and an arteriovenous and Chiari malformation. A PH-tic syndrome (PH plus trigeminal neuralgia) has been diagnosed in a patient with a Chiari I malformation.

4.4.5 Investigations

One of the most important investigations in PH is the positive response to a therapeutic trial of indometacin. As with CH, blood tests are not used routinely, unless there are signs suggestive of an underlying disorder. Neuroimaging should be performed even in patients with typical attacks, as even these can be secondary to a structural lesion.

4.5 SUNCT

SUNCT and SUNA were thought to be extremely rare, with 50 cases of SUNCT published prior to 2003. However, there have been further case reports since then, as well as a large series of 43 patients with SUNCT and nine with SUNA, published in 2006. A recent epidemiological study found two SUNCT-like syndromes in a population of 1838 patients. SUNCT affects men more than women, although it seems that in SUNA the male:female ratio is reversed.

4.5.1 Phenotype

SUNCT is characterized by unilateral pain that is stabbing or throbbing in quality, and is severe. There should be at least 20 attacks, lasting for 5–240 s, and ipsilateral conjunctival injection and lacrimation should be present. SUNCT may be considered the majority subset of SUNA, in which there may be cranial autonomic symptoms other than conjunctival injection and lacrimation, or indeed only one of those symptoms may be present (Table 4.2).

The IHS describes the site of pain in SUNCT as unilateral orbital, supraorbital, or temporal, although the pain may be experienced anywhere in the head. Attacks may take on different characteristics: single stabs, which are usually short-lived, groups of stabs, or a longer attack comprised of many stabs between which the pain does not resolve to normal, thus giving a 'saw-tooth' phenomenon with attacks lasting for many minutes (Figure 4.1).

Important clinical characteristics of SUNCT include triggerability of attacks to cutaneous stimuli such as touching the face, chewing, talking, or cold wind on the face, or other stimuli such as movement of the neck or bright lights. These are more prevalent in SUNCT, for which 74% of patients reported triggering, than in SUNA (22%). Other important features include a lack of refractory period between attacks. Up to 58% of patients are agitated with the attacks, which is a feature of TACs. SUNCT/SUNA may be associated with migrainous symptoms such as nausea, photophobia, or phonophobia, but the aura is not typically a feature.

Patients may suffer from episodic or chronic SUNCT. The chronic form predominates in SUNCT (63%) and SUNA (89%).

Table 4.2 Associated cranial autonomic symptoms (% of cohort)

	CH*	PH†	SUNCT‡	SUNA§
No. in cohort	230	21	43	9
Conjunctival injection	77	57	100	22
Lacrimation	91	80	100	44 (contra-lateral in 1 case)
Nasal blockage	75	57	40	22
Rhinorrhoea	72	47	53	22
Eyelid oedema	74	42	49	11
Ptosis	74	47	51	33
Facial flushing		57	9	11
Sweating: unilateral or bilateral			7	11
Other		‡	9	33

By definition, 100% of patients with SUNCT had both conjunctival injection and lacrimation, and no patients with SUNA had both.

* After Bahra *et al.* (2002a).

† Cittadini and Goadsby (2006).

‡ After Cohen *et al.* (2006b).

§ Includes forehead and facial sweating, mydriasis, aural fullness and swelling (Cittadini and Goadsby 2006).

Figure 4.1 The three types of attack in SUNCT/SUNA

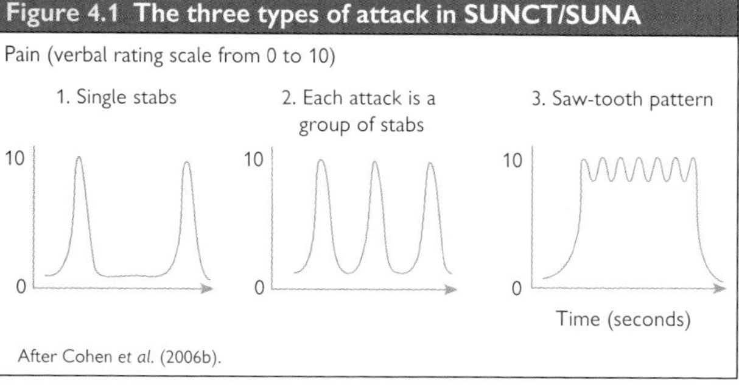

After Cohen *et al.* (2006b).

4.5.2 **Examination**

Generally the neurological examination is normal in primary SUNCT, but there are reports of some trigeminal sensory disturbance.

4.5.3 Diagnosis

As the attacks of SUNCT can vary in length between a few seconds for the single stab, up to many minutes or even hours for the groups of stabs or saw-tooth attacks, the differential diagnosis includes CH, PH, and even trigeminal neuralgia (TN). There is interictal pain in 47% of patients with SUNCT and in 22% of those with SUNA, and in these cases hemicrania continua (HC) enters the differential diagnosis as well. It is often useful to ask the patient to draw a diagram of their attack; a long attack may be mistaken for CH or PH until the 'saw-tooth' element is recognized as SUNCT.

Minimal or no cranial autonomic symptoms and a clear refractory period to triggering are useful pointers to a diagnosis of TN compared with SUNCT/SUNA.

SUNCT can coexist with migraine, with 50% of patients with SUNCT having migrainous biology, which is higher than the 11–15% migraine prevalence in the general population. In some patients the background interictal pain in SUNCT may be attributable to migrainous biology and an analgesic overuse syndrome. There is also a report of a family association of SUNCT.

4.5.4 Secondary/symptomatic SUNCT

Although SUNCT and SUNA are generally primary syndromes, they are proportionately more likely to be symptomatic to underlying pathology than the other TACs (Table 4.3).

Secondary SUNCT and SUNA are typically seen with either posterior fossa or pituitary gland lesions, although local lesions can also cause these syndromes (Figure 4.2).

4.5.5 Investigations

It is recommended that a brain MRI with pituitary views and blood tests for pituitary function should be a minimal work-up for SUNCT/SUNA.

In terms of therapeutic trials, SUNCT may be differentiated from CH by the lack of response to oxygen, and from PH by the lack of response to indometacin. One study showed a striking response of patients with SUNCT and SUNA to intravenous lidocaine.

Table 4.3 Secondary/symptomatic TACs

	Pituitary	Posterior fossa	Vascular	Post-traumatic
CH	+	+	+	+
PH	+	+	+	+
SUNCT	++	++	+	+
SUNA		+	+	

Figure 4.2 Symptomatic/secondary SUNCT/SUNA

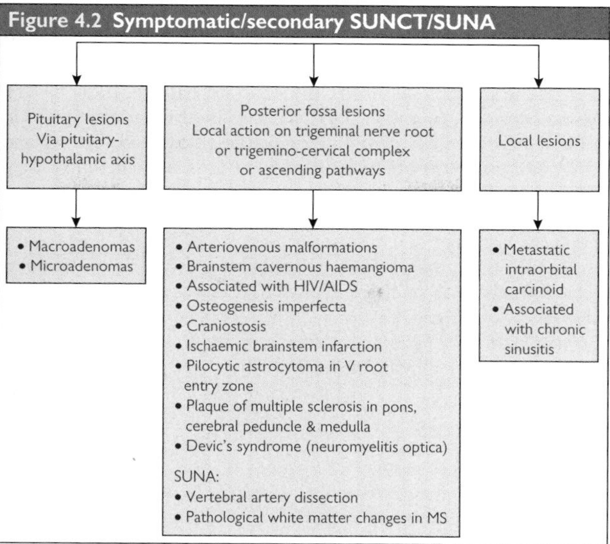

4.6 Hemicrania continua

HC is, as the name suggests, a syndrome of continual pain on one side of the head. The pain may have a moderate background component with exacerbations of severe pain characteristically lasting for hours to days at a time. It may be associated with ipsilateral cranial autonomic symptoms and migrainous features such as nausea and photophobia. HC is characterized neither as a TAC nor as migraine, but it shares features of both syndromes (Headache Classification Committee of The International Headache Society 2004). Its characteristic response to indometacin may link it to PH. Functional imaging work has shown that the activation in HC is both in the region of the posterior hypothalamus, such as in TACs, and in the dorsal rostral pons, such as in migraine.

4.7 Summary

The TACs are stereotyped syndromes that share the features of unilateral, severe or excruciating attacks of pain which are mainly orbital, retro-orbital, or temporal. They are associated mainly with ipsilateral cranial autonomic symptoms, and other features such as agitation. The difference between the TACs can be elucidated from the history: PH attacks are shorter and more frequent than CH attacks, and SUNCT/SUNA attacks are shorter and more numerous still. Long saw-tooth attacks of SUNCT and SUNA may be confused with PH or CH, and the shortest SUNCT/SUNA attacks may be mistaken for first division trigeminal neuralgia. SUNCT makes up the majority subset of SUNA, where SUNCT has both conjunctival injection and tearing, and SUNA has one or the other, but not both.

Examination in these syndromes is generally normal. These are mostly primary headache syndromes, but they can be secondary to underlying structural lesions, especially in SUNCT/SUNA, where the lesions may be in the pituitary or posterior fossa. As more patients are recognized with so-called 'typical' TACs, which are in fact symptomatic of underlying pathology, the recommendation is now to perform brain imaging in all patients with TACs, and blood tests for pituitary function in SUNCT/SUNA.

Key references

Antonaci F, Sjaastad O (1989). Chronic paroxysmal hemicrania (CPH): a review of the clinical manifestations. *Headache* **29**, 648–56.

Bahra A, May A and Goadsby PJ (2002a). Cluster headache: a prospective clinical study in 230 patients with diagnostic implications. *Neurology* **58**, 354–61.

Bahra A, May A and Goadsby PJ (2002b). Cluster headache: a prospective clinical study with diagnostic implications. *Neurology* **58**, 354–61.

Boes CJ and Dodick DW (2002). Refining the clinical spectrum of chronic paroxysmal hemicrania: a review of 74 patients. *Headache* **42**, 699–708.

Cittadini E and Goadsby PJ (2006). Revisiting the International Headache Society criteria for paroxysmal hemicrania: a series of 21 patients. *Cephalalgia* **26**, 1401–2.

Cohen A (2007a). Short-lasting unilateral neuralgiform headache attacks with conjunctival injection and tearing. *Cephalalgia* **27**, 824–32.

Cohen AS, Matharu MS and Goadsby PJ (2006a). Paroxysmal hemicrania in a family. *Cephalalgia* **26**, 486–8.

Cohen AS, Matharu MS and Goadsby PJ (2006b). Short-lasting unilateral neuralgiform headache attacks with conjunctival injection and tearing (SUNCT) or cranial autonomic features (SUNA)—a prospective clinical study of SUNCT and SUNA. *Brain* **129**, 2746–60.

Cohen AS, Matharu MS and Goadsby PJ (2007b). Short-lasting unilateral neuralgiform headache attacks with conjunctival injection and tearing (SUNCT). *Cephalagia* **27**, 824–32.

Favier I, van Vliet JA. Roon KI *et al.* (2007). Trigeminal autonomic cephalgias due to structural lesions: a review of 31 cases. *Arch Neurol* **64**, 25–31.

Goadsby PJ, Cohen AS and Matharu MS (2007). Trigeminal autonomic cephalalgias: diagnosis and treatment. *Curr Neurol Neurosci Rep* **7**, 117–25.

Headache Classification Committee of The International Headache Society (2004). Classification and diagnostic criteria for headache disorders, cranial neuralgias and facial pain (second edition). *Cephalalgia* **24**, 1–160.

Levy MJ, Matharu MS, Meeran K, Powell M and Goadsby PJ (2005). The clinical characteristics of headache in patients with pituitary tumours. *Brain* **128**, 1921–30.

Maggioni F, Palmieri A, Viaro F, Mainardi F and Zanchin G (2007). Menstrual paroxysmal hemicrania, a possible new entity? *Cephalalgia* **27**, 1085–7.

Manzoni GC, Lambru G and Torelli P (2006). Head trauma and cluster headache. *Curr Pain Headache Rep* **10**, 130–6.

Matharu MS, Cohen AS, Boes CJ and Goadsby PJ (2003). Short-lasting unilateral neuralgiform headache with conjunctival injection and tearing syndrome: a review. *Curr Pain Headache Rep* **7**, 308–18.

Russell MB (2007). Genetics in primary headaches. *J Headache Pain* **8**, 190–5.

Schurks M, Kurth T, de Jesus J, Jonjic M, Rosskopf D and Diener HC (2006). Cluster headache: clinical presentation, lifestyle features, and medical treatment. *Headache* **46**, 1246–54.

Sjaastad O and Bakketeig LS (2003). Cluster headache prevalence. Vaga study of headache epidemiology. *Cephalalgia* **23**, 528–33.

Sjaastad O and Bakketeig LS (2007). The rare, unilateral headaches. Vaga study of headache epidemiology. *J Headache Pain* **8**, 19–27.

Chapter 5

Secondary headaches

Julio Pascual

Key points

- There are numerous causes of secondary headache.
- Serious secondary headache should be excluded by evaluating headache alarms.
- The next step is to identify or exclude other secondary headaches versus primary headaches.
- For some secondary headaches, the accompanying symptoms and signs make the underlying diagnosis obvious.
- For other secondary headaches, headache may be the main or even the only symptom, and can mimic any primary headache.

5.1 **Introduction**

Headache is a symptom that can have many causes. When evaluating a patient with a headache, the first task is to exclude a serious secondary headache. This decision is based on the history and the general medical and neurological examinations.

The next step in the differential diagnosis is to identify or exclude other secondary headaches versus primary headaches. For most secondary headaches, the characteristics of the headache itself do not contribute much to help establish the cause.

The causes of secondary headaches are numerous (Table 5.1). Once sinister headaches have been excluded, there are two facts to bear in mind in clinical practice. First, in patients consulting for headache, primary headaches are more frequent than secondary headaches, even in patients with alarm symptoms. Second, for the most common secondary headaches, such as alcohol overuse, infections, or trauma, the aetiology is obvious. For a number of secondary headaches, for instance headache due to an established stroke, headache itself is not the diagnostic symptom.

Table 5.1 Main diagnostic alarms in headache evaluation

Alarm	Serious causes	Common causes
HA begins at age >50 years	Temporal arteritis Mass lesion	Tension-type HA
Sudden-onset HA	Subarachnoid bleeding Pituitary apoplexy Bleed into a mass lesion	Primary exertional HA
Accelerating pattern of HA	Mass lesion Subdural haematoma	MOH
HA with fever	Meningitis Encephalitis Abscess	Systemic infection
Focal neurological signs/symptoms	Stroke Mass lesion Vascular malformation	Migraine aura
HA plus papilloedema	Mass lesion	Idiopathic intracranial hypertension (pseudo-tumour cerebri)
HA plus red eye	Acute glaucoma	TAC

HA, headache; MOH, medication overuse headache; TAC, trigeminal autonomic cephalalgia.

Therefore, in clinical practice, differential diagnosis of secondary headaches concentrates on those secondary headaches that express headache as the main or even isolated symptom, which could mimic any of the most frequent primary headaches (Figure 5.1). This chapter focuses on these headaches and on secondary headaches that show a specific headache pattern.

5.2 Headache attributed to vascular disorders

5.2.1 Headache attributed to transient ischaemic attacks

Headache appears in around 30% of transient ischaemic attacks (TIAs), most commonly in basilar rather than carotid TIAs, and is rarely a prominent phenomenon. The differential diagnosis with the first episode of migraine aura can be difficult. Clues favouring a diagnosis of headache due to TIA include: old age, acute onset, and the absence of positive visual symptoms (e.g. scintillating scotoma).

Figure 5.1 Algorithm for headache diagnosis

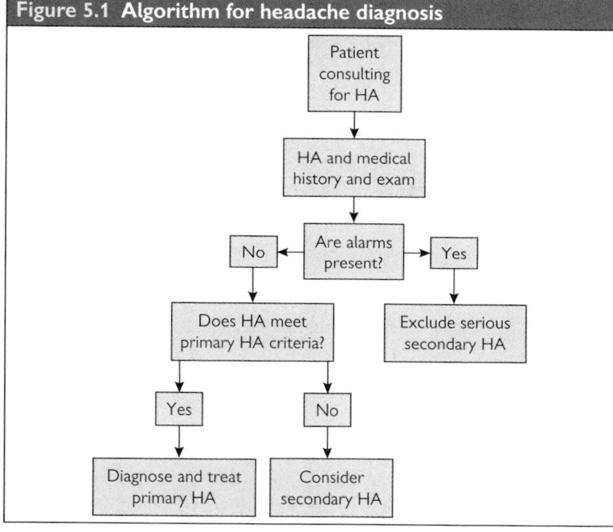

5.2.2 **Headache attributed to subarachnoid haemorrhage**

Subarachnoid haemorrhage is a neurosurgical emergency. Typically, acute headache occurs with exercise and is accompanied by vomiting, loss of consciousness, and nuchal rigidity. In some patients, severe subarachnoid haemorrhage is preceded by small leaks manifesting as isolated headaches. The key to diagnosis is the abrupt onset. Even so, 80% of these patients will be diagnosed as having primary exertional headache (Figure 5.2). Any patient with headache of abrupt onset must be evaluated immediately to exclude subarachnoid haemorrhage. Ancillary examinations must include computed tomography (CT), without contrast or flair magnetic resonance imaging (MRI) sequences, and, in case of doubt, a lumbar puncture.

5.2.3 **Headache attributed to giant cell arteritis**

Headache is the first symptom in 90% of patients with temporal arteritis (Figure 5.3), whereas the presence of other characteristic symptoms of this entity (polymyalgia rheumatica, jaw claudication) is more variable and delayed.

Therefore, in any *de novo* persisting headache in a patient over 60 years of age, giant cell arteritis must be ruled out as the short-term risk of blindness (and other serious complications) is high. Erythrocyte sedimentation rate and C-reactive protein concentration are crucial,

Figure 5.2 Diagnostic approach for activity-related headaches

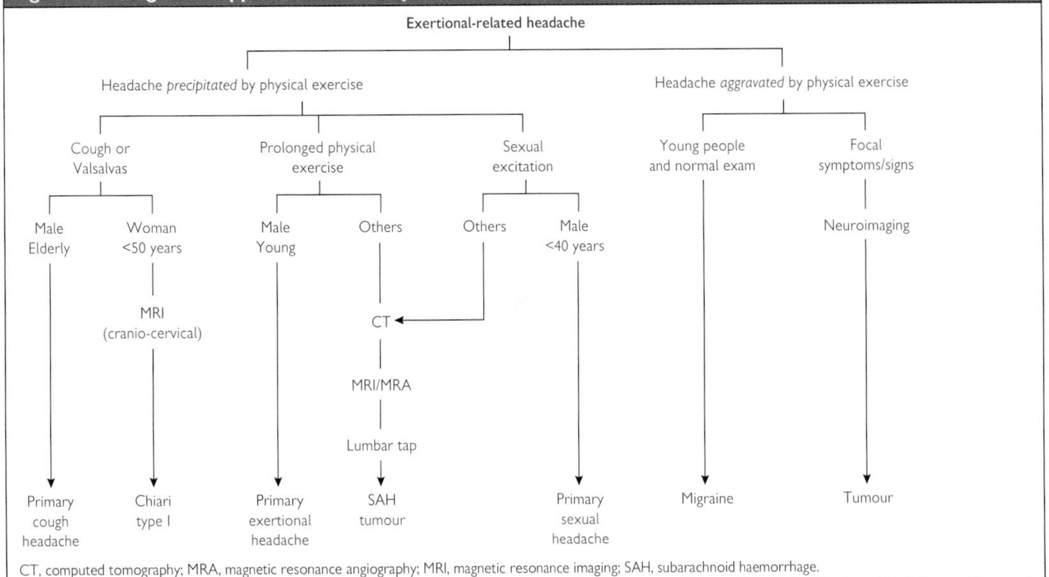

CT, computed tomography; MRA, magnetic resonance angiography; MRI, magnetic resonance imaging; SAH, subarachnoid haemorrhage.

Figure 5.3 A thickened and painful temporal artery in a 79-year-old man consulting because of recent-onset headache due to giant cell arteritis

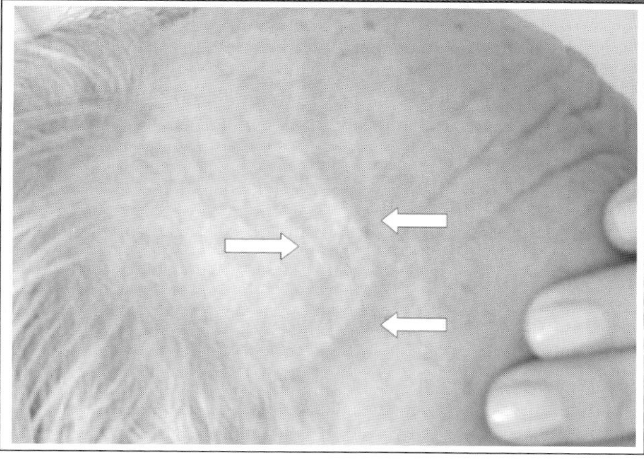

as both are clearly raised in 95% of cases. Duplex scanning of the temporal arteries may visualize the thickened arterial wall (as a halo on axial sections) and may help to select the site for the biopsy. If biopsy is negative but clinical suspicion remains high, resolution of headache within 3 days of high-dose steroid treatment is of great diagnostic help.

5.2.4 **Headache attributed to arterial dissection**

Headache, with or without neck pain, is the most frequent symptom of arterial cervical dissection (55–100% of cases). Headache is usually unilateral, ipsilateral to the dissected artery, and has no specific pattern—it can mimic other headaches, such as migraine, cluster headaches, or subarachnoid haemorrhage. Associated symptoms are frequent: signs of cerebral or retinal ischaemia and focal signs. A painful Horner's syndrome, or a painful tinnitus of sudden onset, is highly suggestive of carotid dissection. Vertebral dissection produces neck and occipital pain. The abrupt onset and association of brainstem ischaemic symptoms could prevent confusion with migraine, but differential diagnosis with basilar migraine is sometimes difficult. Headache usually precedes the onset of ischaemic signs. Diagnostic examinations include duplex scanning, magnetic resonance angiography (MRA) or helical CT, and, if necessary, conventional angiography.

5.2.5 **Headache attributed to cerebral venous thrombosis**

Headache is the most frequent inaugural symptom of cerebral venous thrombosis (CVT) and is its most common symptom (>80% cases). Headache in CVT can mimic any kind of headache, although it is usually diffuse, progressive, and associated with other signs of intracranial hypertension. Typically, focal seizures/neurological deficits appear days or a few weeks after the onset of headache (Figure 5.4). In the presence of an underlying prothrombotic condition, any new persistent headache must raise the suspicion of CVT. MRI plus MRA is usually enough to confirm or rule out the diagnosis.

5.3 **Headache attributed to nonvascular intracranial disorder**

5.3.1 **Headache attributed to high or low cerebrospinal fluid pressure**

Headache is the main symptom of both high and low cerebrospinal fluid (CSF) pressure syndromes. Headache due to increased intracranial CSF pressure is typically progressive, diffuse, and aggravates with coughing or straining. Papilloedema and VIth nerve palsy can be seen on examination.

Figure 5.4 MRI showing a fresh clot (arrow) in a patient with headache due to superior sagittal sinus thrombosis

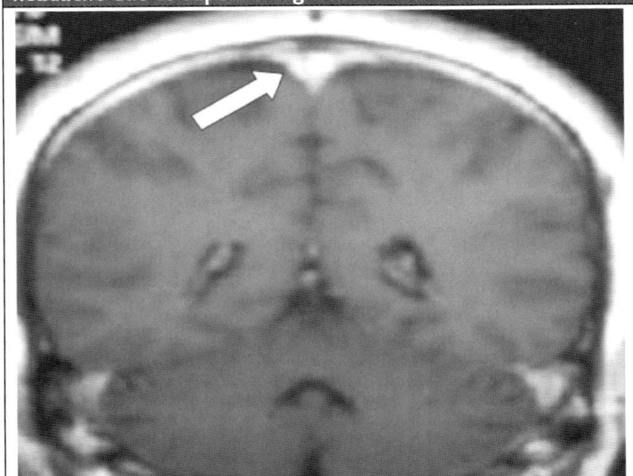

Brain tumours represent a small minority of the causes of headache, although they are a major concern. Except for children and middle line tumours leading to hydrocephalus, such as colloid cyst of the third ventricle or fourth ventricle tumours, headache is rarely an isolated presenting manifestation of brain neoplasms, which typically begin as seizures or focal symptoms. Headache, mostly with other symptoms, appears at the initial diagnosis in approximately one-third of patients with brain tumours and develops in the course of the disease in two-thirds. Headache awakening the patient from sleep or present on awakening and associated with vomiting is a frequent characteristic of brain tumours, but also may occur in migraineurs.

Headache is the main clinical symptom of so-called pseudotumour cerebri or idiopathic intracranial hypertension (Figure 5.5). This diagnosis should be suspected in young obese women with headache, papilloedema, and normal findings on neuroimaging.

Figure 5.5 Papilloedema due to idiopathic intracranial hypertension

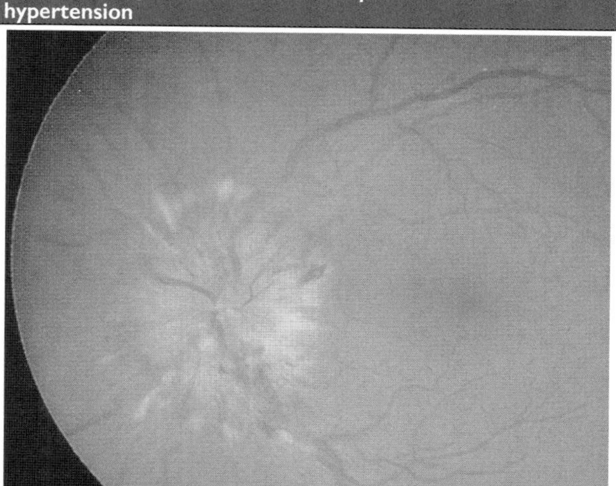

Other symptoms of this syndrome are monocular, transient (seconds) visual obscurations, double vision, and tinnitus. Diagnosis is confirmed by finding an increased CSF pressure and a normal CSF chemistry in the lumbar puncture.

Headache due to low CSF pressure is very characteristic and can be suspected from the clinical interview. These patients, usually young and thin women, complain of orthostatic headache, that is, their headache worsens (or begins) within 15 min after sitting or standing, and improves (or disappears) immediately after lying. The headache can be accompanied by neck stiffness, tinnitus, photophobia, nausea, or even horizontal double vision, due to VIth nerve paresis. In most of these patients, headache follows lumbar puncture or epidural anaesthesia, although there are spontaneous cases. Diagnosis can be confirmed by pachymeningeal enhancement on MRI (Figure 5.6).

5.3.2 **Headache due to Chiari malformation**

Headache precipitated by cough or other Valsalva maneuvers can be primary or secondary. Two-thirds of headaches precipitated by cough are secondary, and most of these are due to a Chiari type I malformation (Figure 5.7).

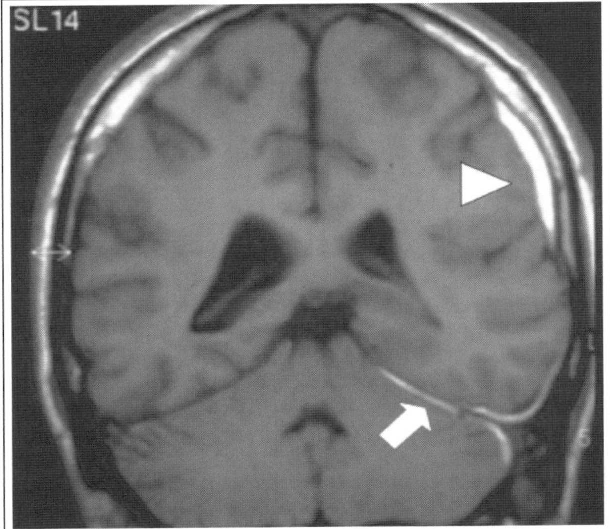

Figure 5.6 MRI with gadolinium showing pachymeningeal enhancement (arrow) and a small subdural haematoma (arrowhead) in a patient with orthostatic headache due to spontaneous low CSF pressure.

Figure 5.7 MRI showing tonsillar descent (arrow) under the Chamberlain line (dotted line) in a patient with cough headache due to Chiari type I malformation

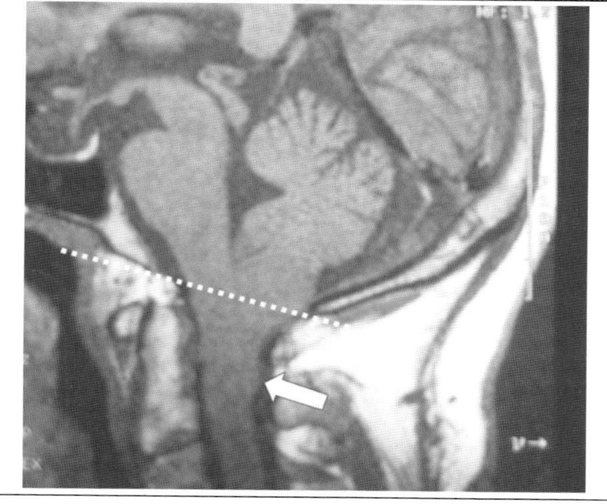

Clues for diagnosis in primary cough headache are old age, no other associated neurological symptoms/signs, and response to indometacin. Craniocervical MRI is therefore mandatory in these patients, mainly if they are young, if there are posterior fossa symptoms/signs, and if there is no response to indometacin. The diagnostic approach to headaches that develop following physical effort is illustrated in Figure 5.2.

5.3.3 **Headache due to syndrome of headache and neurological deficits with CSF lymphocytosis (HaNDL)**

The clinical picture of this syndrome, also called pseudomigraine with pleocytosis, is of one to more than ten discrete episodes of transient neurological deficits lasting for hours, accompanied or followed by moderate to severe headache. The usual neurological manifestations are unilateral sensory and/or motor symptoms and aphasia. Brainstem dysfunction and visual symptoms are rare. The episodes may recur for several weeks (up to 3 months) and patients are asymptomatic between episodes. A lumbar tap discloses CSF lymphocytosis and increased levels of CSF protein. Microbiological studies, CT, and MRI are normal. Electroencephalography and brain single-photon emission computed tomography (SPECT) can disclose focal abnormalities during episodes (Figure 5.8). The syndrome is benign and self-limiting.

Figure 5.8 **Brain SPECT showing left occipital hypometabolism (arrow) in a patient with pseudomigraine with pleocytosis**

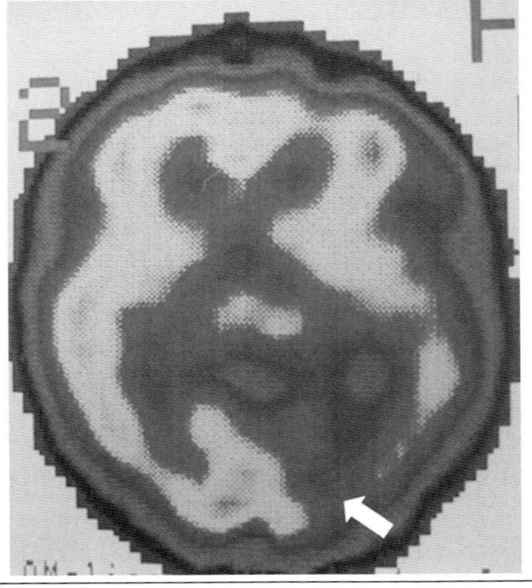

5.4 **Headache attributed to a substance or its withdrawal**

5.4.1 **Medication overuse headache**

In clinical practice, many patients with the alarm symptom of accelerating headache pattern suffer from chronic daily headache (headache for more than 15 days per month of more than 4 h in duration) with overuse of acute medications, that is, consumption of symptomatic medication for more than 2 days per week. Typically these patients have a previous history of episodic migraine or tension-type headache. Attacks increase in frequency over a number of years or decades until a pattern of daily/almost daily headache develops, usually around 40 years of age.

In chronic migraine, the nature of headache changes over time; pain becomes mild to moderate rather than moderate to severe, and the associated symptoms become less frequent and severe. Over time, patients develop a daily headache pattern consisting of a background continuous headache, with superimposed bouts of migraine attacks. Transformation from episodic to chronic migraine does not necessarily mean that it is secondary to medication overuse, although this should be considered in all patients presenting with a pattern of chronic migraine. It may also reflect the natural history of the disease, or may be related to co-morbid depression and/or anxiety, or to a combination of all these factors.

5.5 Headache attributed to disorder of the cranium, neck, eyes, ears, nose, sinuses, teeth, mouth, or other facial/cranial structure

These disorders are frequently regarded as the commonest causes of headache. Non-specific headache is usually attributed to spondylosis, chronic sinusitis, temporomandibular joint disorders, or refractive errors of the eyes, but these disorders are just as widespread among individuals who do not suffer from headaches.

5.5.1 Cervicogenic headache

As many headaches originate in the cervical regions, disorders of the cervical spine have been regarded as a common cause of headache. Radiological evidence of cervical spondylosis is not a satisfactory explanation for a headache, because it can be found with equal prevalence in age-matched headache-free subjects.

True cervicogenic headache is, in principle, a strict unilateral headache. Otherwise, this headache will be confused with tension-type headache or migraine without aura. The duration of the solitary attack—or an exacerbation—varies from a few hours to a few weeks. In the initial phase, the headache is usually episodic; later, it frequently becomes chronic and fluctuating. Symptoms and signs referable to the neck are essential, such as a reduced range of motion in the neck or mechanical precipitation of attacks. 'Migrainous' symptoms such as nausea and photophobia are, when present, generally not marked. A positive response to appropriate anaesthetic blockades is essential.

The scarcity of autonomic symptoms and signs distinguishes this headache from cluster headache, as do other features, such as the temporal pattern, severity, and female preponderance. Hemicrania continua and cervicogenic headache have many traits in common as far as clinical manifestations and developmental patterns are concerned. Both disorders frequently begin with a remitting headache, which may eventually develop into a chronic type. However, precipitation mechanisms are not an integral part of hemicrania continua, and the response to indometacin is a decisive factor in the differential diagnosis.

5.5.2 Headache attributed to rhinosinusitis

The diagnosis of headache due to acute sinusitis is easy on clinical grounds. Chronic sinusitis is not a cause of headache. Many of these patients fulfil the criteria for migraine without aura.

5.5.3 Headache attributed to acute glaucoma

Acute glaucoma in adults can result in severe eye and supraorbital pain (Figure 5.9). Attacks may occur at night and resemble migraine, and can be accompanied by visual symptoms. Glaucoma must be suspected in patients with *de novo*, strictly unilateral, pain in the eye region, mainly if they are older than 50 years. The affected globe may be hard on palpation, the cornea steamy, and the ipsilateral pupil is usually dilated. Ophthalmological examination confirms the diagnosis.

Figure 5.9 Right conjunctival injection and dilated pupil in a patient with acute glaucoma who consulted due to a right periocular headache and blurred vision

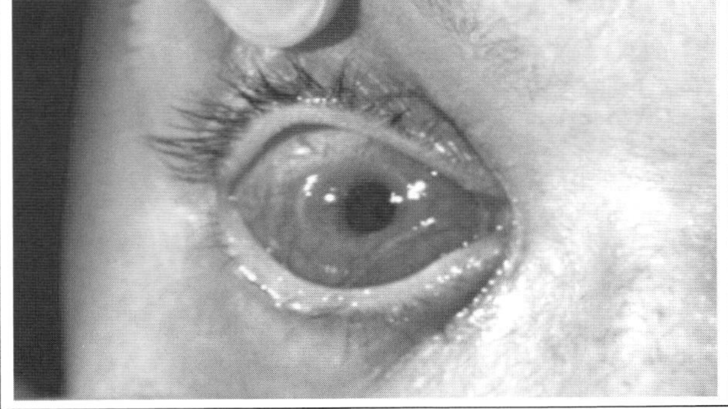

Key references

Goadsby PJ, Silberstein SD and Dodick D (2005). *Chronic Daily Headache for Clinicians*. BC Decker, Hamilton.

Gómez-Aranda F, Cañadillas F, Martí-Massó JF *et al.* (1996). Pseudomigraine with temporary neurological symptoms and lymphocytic pleocytosis. A report of 50 cases. *Brain* **120**, 1105–13.

Headache Classification Subcommittee of the International Headache Society (2004). The International Classification of Headache Disorders, 2nd edition. *Cephalalgia* **24(suppl 1)**, 1–160.

Olesen J, Goadsby PJ, Ramadan NM, Tfelt-Hansen P and Welch KMA (2006). *The Headaches*, 3rd edn. Lippincott Williams & Wilkins, Philadelphia.

Pascual J, Iglesias F, Oterino A, Vázquez-Barquero A and Berciano J (1996). Cough, exertional, and sexual headaches: an analysis of 72 benign and symptomatic cases. *Neurology* **46**, 1520–4.

Schmidt WA, Kraft HE, Vorpahl K, Völker L and Gromnica-Ihle EJ (1997). Color duplex ultrasonography in the diagnosis of temporal arteritis. *N Engl J Med* **337**, 1336–42.

Part 2
Pathophysiology

Chapter 6

Migraine

Messoud Ashina

Key points

- Migraine is a neurovascular disorder with a genetic component.
- Migraine aura is caused by cortical spreading depression.
- Migraine headache is due to activation of perivascular nociceptors and subsequent plastic changes in the central nervous system.
- Nitric oxide and calcitonin gene-related peptide play a key role in pathophysiology.

6.1 Genetics

Migraine is a group of familial disorders with a genetic component. Familial hemiplegic migraine (FHM) is a rare, dominantly inherited, subtype of migraine with aura characterized by attacks of migraine, with and without aura, and hemiparesis, International Headache Classification (IHCD-II).

Three types of FHM have so far been identified genetically (Table 6.1). FHM type 1 (FHM-1) is caused by missense mutations in the *CACNA1A* gene on chromosome 19p13, encoding the α1A subunit of calcium channels, FHM type 2 (FHM-2) is caused by mutations in the *ATP1A2* gene encoding the α_2 subunit of a Na^+, K^+ ATPase, and FHM type 3 (FHM-3) is caused by mutations in the *SCN1A* gene encoding a neuronal voltage-gated sodium channel. FHM-1 and FHM-2 are caused by several different mutations. However, only one heterozygote mutation has been described in FHM-3.

An epidemiological study of a population based FHM cohort showed that 65% of patients with FHM had migraine with aura (MA) and/or migraine without aura (MO). It has been reported that MA and MO are not associated with any of the known FHM mutations. The identification of the mutated FHM genes stimulated interest in the link between genotype and phenotype using both molecular studies and animal models. Interestingly, *CACNA1A* knock-in mice homozygous for the human FHM R192Q mutation showed increased susceptibility to cortical spreading depression. Knock-in mice with the FHM-2 and FHM-3 mutations have not yet been developed.

Table 6.1 Familial hemiplegic migraine (FHM)			
Name	**Gene symbol**	**Locus**	**Protein name**
FHM-1	*CACNA1A*	19p13	Voltage-dependent P/Q-type calcium channel subunit α1A
FHM-2	*ATP1A2*	1q21-q23	Sodium/potassium-transporting ATPase subunit α2
FHM-3	*SCN1A*	2q24	Sodium channel protein type 1 subunit α

ATPase, adenosine triphosphatase.
Sources: De Fusco M, Marconi R, Silvestri L, Atorino L, Rampoldi L, Morgante L, Ballabio A, Aridon P, Casari G (2003). Haploinsufficiency of ATP1A2 encoding the Na+/K+ pump

The functional consequences of FHM mutations in humans, however, are not fully clarified, and the potential species differences should be considered. Recently, an interesting approach has been introduced to elucidate the functional consequences of FHM mutations. Patients with known genetic mutations were exposed to known migraine triggers such as glyceryl trinitrate (GTN). Hansen *et al.* examined genotyped FHM-1 and FHM-2 patients using the GTN model of migraine, and found that these mutations were not associated with hypersensitivity to activation of the nitric oxide–cyclic guanosine monophosphate pathway. These data suggest that neurobiological pathways responsible for migraine headache in MO and MA may be distinct from the pathways responsible for migraine headache in FHM.

6.2 **Aura**

There is now a common consensus that the aura is caused by cortical spreading depression (CSD). CSD was first demonstrated as an animal experimental phenomenon in 1944 by Leao, who also suggested that it was relevant to migraine. It is characterized by shifts in cortical steady-state potential, transient increases in potassium, nitric oxide, and glutamate concentrations, and transient increases in cortical blood flow, followed by sustained decreases. In the 1980s a series of studies of human regional cerebral blood flow (rCBF) during MA showed pathognomonic changes in rCBF typical of CSD. The aura was associated with an initial hyperaemic phase followed by reduced cortical blood flow, which moved across the cortex (spreading oligaemia). Posterior cortical blood flow was reduced by 17–35% and spread anteriorly at 2–3 mm/min. Reduced cortical blood flow persisted for 30 min to 6 h, then slowly returned to baseline or increased. The rates of progression of spreading oligaemia were similar to those of migrainous scotoma and CSD, suggesting that they were related. It is important to notice that headache often begins while cortical blood flow is reduced. This indicates that headache is not caused by simple reflex vasodilatation. Newer techniques such as functional magnetic resonance imaging have lately confirmed rCBF changes during human migraine attacks that are very similar to CSD. These results led to the development of tonabersat, a compound with no known binding site, but with the ability to block CSD efficiently in animal experiments. This compound failed in the acute studies, but recently showed a tendency for a better response than placebo in a migraine prevention trial.

The relation between CSD and headache in MA is a matter of intense debate. Animal experiments have shown that CSD may cause activation of the caudal portion of the trigeminal nucleus in the brainstem. At the same time, collateral axons of activated neurones in the trigeminal ganglion release proinflammatory peptides in the meninges and their vessels, leading to a local inflammatory reaction. However, this plausible biological mechanism for aura-generating headache is in contrast to clinical observations; for example, aura and headache may occur on the same side, aura without headache is well recognized, and aura does not necessarily precede headache, that is, aura may occur with the onset of headache or even after hours or days of headache. Thus, the relationship between aura and migraine headache is not fully clarified.

6.3 **Headache**

Migraine headache is believed to be generated by activity in cranial perivascular afferents, in particular from dural vessels (Figure 6.1).

Moskowitz's neurogenic inflammation animal model of migraine suggested that during migraine an unidentified stimulus prompts the trigeminal nerve fibres surrounding the blood vessels to release stored peptides, such as calcitonin gene-related peptide (CGRP) and substance P, and subsequently causes an aseptic inflammation of the blood vessels. It has been shown that triptans, dihydroergotamine, and non-steroidal inflammatory agents prevent the stimulation-induced leakage of plasma proteins within the dura mater. The neurogenic inflammation model has been used as a model of migraine to test the antimigraine efficacy of drugs without causing vasoconstriction. Several such substances were found, including CP-122,288, a highly potent inhibitor of neurogenic plasma extravasation in animal models. All of these compounds could block neurogenic inflammation, but failed to relieve migraine in clinical trials.

In the past two decades, there has been increased focus on possible brainstem mechanisms of migraine, the role of central sensitization, nitric oxide (NO), and CGRP in the pathophysiology of migraine.

Figure 6.1 Pathophysiology of migraine

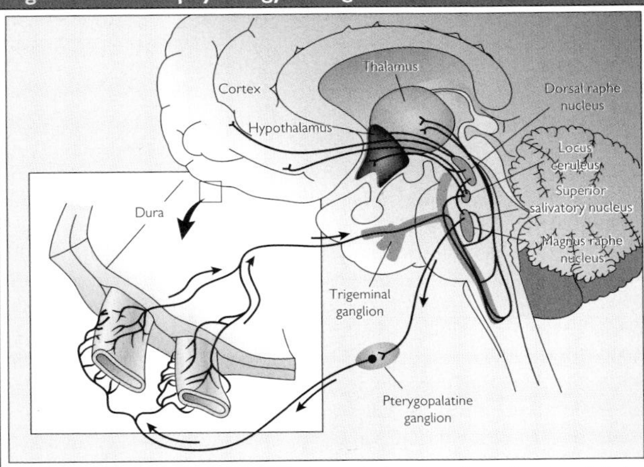

The key pathways for migraine are the trigeminovascular input from the meningeal vessels that passes through the trigeminal ganglion and synapses on second-order neurones in the trigemiocervical complex. These neurones, in turn, project through the quintothalamic tract and, after decussating in the brainstem, form synapses with neurones in the thalamus. There is a reflex connection between neurones in the pons in the superior salivatory nucleus; this results in a cranial parasympathetic outflow that is mediated through the pterygopalatine, otic, and carotid ganglia.

Brainstem activation occurs in MO. By use of positron emission tomography, patients with right-sided migraine headache showed increased rCBF in the left brainstem. Sumatriptan relieved the headache and associated symptoms, but did not normalize rCBF in the brainstem, suggesting that activation is caused by factors other than, or in addition to, increased activity of the endogenous antinociceptive system. Brainstem activation was also reported during GTN-induced migraine.

NO involvement in migraine has been analysed in a series of provocation experiments using nitroglycerin/glyceryl trinitrate (GTN) as a NO donor. It was first shown that infusion of GTN causes a more intense immediate headache during the infusion in patients with migraine than in normal subjects, and, more importantly, also leads to a delayed headache. This delayed headache was maximal around 6–7 h after the infusion, and delayed headache has the characteristics of typical attacks of MO. A non-selective nitric oxide synthase (NOS)

Figure 6.1 adapted from Goadsby PJ, Lipton RB, Ferrari MD (2002). Migraine—current understanding and treatment. *N Engl J Med* **346**: 257–70, with permission from the Publishing Division of the Massachusetts Medical Society.

inhibitor, N^G-monomethyl-L-arginine (L-NMMA), was effective in treating spontaneous migraine attacks. This suggests that NO is an important offending molecule throughout the duration of a migraine attack. L-NMMA has poor bioavailability, a short duration of action, and blocks endothelial NOS, leading to an increase in systemic blood pressure. Therefore, the pharmaceutical industry developed a selective inducible NOS (iNOS) inhibitor GW274150, which is a highly selective inhibitor of iNOS and offers the potential of anti-inflammatory activity in migraine through a novel mechanism of action. This compound has already entered clinical phase II trials, whereas a selective neuronal NOS (nNOS) inhibitor has entered phase I trial.

Burstein and colleagues showed that inflammatory molecules administered to the dura of rats activate and sensitize peripheral and central trigeminovascular neurones. Moreover, it has been shown that triptans may exert their antimigraine action through presynaptic 5-$HT_{1B/1D}$ receptors in the dorsal horn by blocking synaptic transmission between axon terminals of the peripheral trigemino-vascular neurones and the cell bodies of their central counterparts. Because animal studies suggested an association between increased periorbital skin sensitivity and intracranial pain Burstein *et al.* hypothesized that it may also be present during migraine attacks in humans. The authors subsequently studied patients with migraine during and outside an attack. Cutaneous allodynia was defined as pain resulting from a non-noxious stimulus such as heat, cold, or pressure to normal skin. The major finding of this study was that 79% of patients presented cutaneous allodynia. Interestingly, some of patients reported allodynia in non-cephalic regions. The authors suggested that cutaneous allodynia is either due to sensitization of second-order (extracranial allodynia) and/or third-order (extracranial and non-cephalic allodynia) neurones. Thus, migraineurs may exhibit signs of cutaneous allodynia during attacks, and extracranial hypersensitivity could be a manifestation of central sensitization.

CGRP is a 37-amino-acid neuropeptide, identified in 1982. CGRP immunoreactivity was shown in the trigeminal ganglia. In 1984, an *in vitro* study reported, for the first time, calcium-dependent release of CGRP upon depolarization from trigeminal ganglia. A dense supply of CGRP-containing fibres around the cerebral vessels was reported to originate in the trigeminal ganglion. Furthermore, CGRP innervates human cerebral arteries and is a potent vasodilator of human arteries. It mediates relaxation of these arteries via activation of the CGRP (1) type of receptor. In 1988, Goadsby *et al.* reported that CGRP was released in the extracerebral circulation of humans during thermo-coagulation of trigeminal ganglion. Studies in migraine patients showed an increase in the concentration of CGRP during and outwith migraine attacks. A recent study has challenged these reports, showing no changes in plasma CGRP levels during migraine attacks compared with that outwith attacks. However, recent studies in patients with migraine has provided definitive poof of CGRP involvement in migraine pathogenesis. First, Lassen and colleagues demonstrated that intravenous infusion of CGRP may cause migraine in patients who have migraine attacks. Second, a proof of concept study demonstrated the efficacy of the CGRP receptor antagonist in the treatment of acute migraine attacks. Final proof was recently reported by showing the efficacy of an oral formulation of the CGRP receptor antagonist in the treatment of acute migraine.

6.4 Conclusion

Migraine is a neurovascular disorder in which genetic susceptibility renders the brain in migraineurs more sensitive to a range of trigger factors. The migraine aura is probably caused by CSD. Migraine headache probably results from activation of meningeal and blood vessel nociceptors, and subsequent plastic changes in the central nervous system. The molecular mechanisms triggering migraine aura and headache are unknown. Brainstem activation is probably due to increased activity of the endogenous antinociceptive system. The study of cutaneous allodynia in migraine has provided a link between basic research and clinical studies that importantly contributes to our understanding of mechanisms underlying migraine. CGRP and NO are involved in the pathophysiology of migraine, and antagonism of these molecules may provide a novel principle in the treatment of migraine.

Key references

Burstein R (2001). Deconstructing migraine headache into peripheral and central sensitization. *Pain* **89**, 107–10.

De Fusco M, Marconi R, Silvestri L, Atorino L, Rampoldi L, Morgante L, Ballabio A, Aridon P, Casari G (2003). Haploinsufficiency of ATP1A2 encoding the Na^+/K^+ pump alpha2 subunit associated with familial hemiplegic migraine type 2. *Nat Genet* **33**, 192–6.

Dichgans M, Freilinger T, Eckstein G, Babini E, Lorenz-Depiereux B, Biskup S, Ferrari MD, Herzog J, van den Maagdenberg AM, Pusch M, Strom TM (2005). Mutation in the neuronal voltage-gated sodium channel SCN1A in familial hemiplegic migraine. *Lancet* **366**, 371–7.

Ducros A, Denier C, Joutel A, Cecillon M, Lescoat C, Vahedi K, Darcel F, Vicaut E, Bousser MG, Tournier-Lasserve E. (2001). The clinical spectrum of familial hemiplegic migraine associated with mutations in a neuronal calcium channel. *N Engl J Med* **345**(1): 17–24.

Goadsby PJ, Edvinsson L, Ekman R (1988). Release of vasoactive peptides in the extracerebral circulation of humans and the cat during activation of the trigeminovascular system. *Ann Neurol* **23**, 193–6.

Goadsby PJ (2007). Recent advances in understanding migraine mechanisms, molecules and therapeutics. *Trends Mol Med* **13**, 39–44.

Goadsby PJ, Lipton RB and Ferrari MD (2002). Migraine—current understanding and treatment. *N Engl J Med* **346**, 257–70.

Hansen JM, Thomsen LL, Marconi R, Casari G, Olesen J, Ashina M (2008): Familial hemiplegic migraine type 2 does not share hypersensitivity to nitric oxide with common types of migraine. *Cephalalgia* **28** (4), 367–75.

Hansen JM, Thomsen LL, Olesen J, Ashina M (2008): Familial hemiplegic migraine type 1 shows no hypersensitivity to nitric oxide. *Cephalalgia* **28**, 496–505.

Lassen LH, Ashina M, Christiansen I, Ulrich V and Olesen J (1997). Nitric oxide synthase inhibition in migraine [letter]. *Lancet* **349**, 401–2.

Moskowitz MA (1993). Neurogenic inflammation in the pathophysiology and treatment of migraine. *Neurology* **43**, S16–20.

Olesen J, Friberg L, Olsen TS *et al.* (1990). Timing and topography of cerebral blood flow, aura, and headache during migraine attacks. *Ann Neurol* **28**, 791–8.

Olesen J, Diener HC, Husstedt IW *et al.* (2004). Calcitonin gene-related peptide receptor antagonist BIBN 4096 BS for the acute treatment of migraine. *N Engl J Med* **350**, 1104–10.

Ophoff RA, Terwindt GM, Vergouwe MN, van Eijk R, Oefner PJ, Hoffman SM, Lamerdin JE, Mohrenweiser HW, Bulman DE, Ferrari M, Haan J, Lindhout D, van Ommen GJ, Hofker MH, Ferrari MD, Frants RR (1996): Familial hemiplegic migraine and episodic ataxia type-2 are caused by mutations in the Ca^{2+} channel gene CACNL1A4. *Cell* **87**(3), 543–52.

van den Maagdenberg AM, Haan J, Terwindt GM and Ferrari MD (2007). Migraine: gene mutations and functional consequences. *Curr Opin Neurol* **20**, 299–305.

Weiller C, May A, Limmroth V *et al.* (1995). Brain stem activation in spontaneous human migraine attacks. *Nat Med* **1**, 658–60.

Chapter 7

Tension-type headache

Arnaud Fumal and Jean Schoenen

Key points

- Tension-type headache is an ill-defined and heterogeneous syndrome.
- Peripheral pain mechanisms are most likely to play a role in episodic tension-type headache.
- Central dysnociception seems to be predominant in chronic tension-type headache.
- This chapter summarizes the known pathophysiological features of tension-type headache and proposes a pathogenic model.

7.1 Introduction

Tension-type headache (TTH) is an ill-defined and heterogeneous syndrome, for which diagnosis is based mainly on the absence of features found in other headache types such as migraine. It is thus above all a 'featureless' headache, characterized by nothing but pain in the head. TTH is the most common form of headache, but only chronic TTH (CTTH) that causes headache for 15 or more days per month represents a major health problem with an enormous socio-economic impact.

We have gained much new knowledge on pathophysiological aspects of TTH within the last decade, and are now beginning to understand some of the complex mechanisms leading to this prevalent condition.

7.2 Mechanisms

It still is a matter of debate whether the pain in TTH originates from myofascial tissues or from central mechanisms in the brain. Research progress is hampered by the difficulty in obtaining homogeneous populations of patients, because of the lack of specificity of clinical features and diagnostic criteria.

The present consensus is none the less that peripheral pain mechanisms are most likely to play a role in infrequent episodic TTH

(ETTH) and frequent ETTH, whereas central dysnociception becomes predominant in chronic TTH.

We will summarize below some of the known pathophysiological features and propose a pathogenic model. The data that we will discuss were obtained chiefly from clinical populations of patients with TTH (i.e. in frequent/chronic TTH).

7.2.1 **Myofascial factors**

Muscle activity and metabolism

The level of electromyographic (EMG) activity in pericranial muscle is on average higher in patients with CTTH than in healthy controls, but this is rarely the case if only a few muscles are explored, and there is no correlation whatsoever between EMG levels and the presence or intensity of headache. As a corollary, increased hardness of pericranial muscles has been described in CTTH, but again there is little correlation with headache intensity. During rest or exercise, trapezius muscle lactate levels did not differ between patients with CTTH and healthy volunteers. The exercise-induced increase in trapezius muscle blood flow, however, was blunted in patients, which was interpreted as increased sympathetic vasoconstriction due to hyperexcitable central nervous system neurones. In addition, at trapezius muscle tender points in patients with CTTH there was no increase of inflammatory mediators.

Taken together, these studies do not favour increased activity, or muscular inflammation or disturbed metabolism of pericranial muscles, as important pathogenic factors in CTTH.

Tenderness and pain thresholds

The role of myofascial factors in TTH has been explored by assessing pericranial tenderness on manual palpation or pain detection/tolerance thresholds with a pressure algometer. The results obtained with these methods are not superimposable for methodological reasons. Pressure pain thresholds (PPTs) are usually recorded from one or two cranial locations, mainly the anterior temporal region which is a precise spot with low tenderness on manual palpation in patients with TTH. Tenderness scores on manual palpation are usually summed up from a number of pericranial locations. There is none the less a significant inverse relationship between local tenderness and PPT.

Tenderness on manual palpation is assessed over seven or eight locations on both sides of the cranium, scoring pain between 0 and 3 and summing these scores to obtain a total tenderness score (TTS), which has proved to be reliable. Pericranial tenderness is increased during headache-free intervals and increases further during the headache in most patients with TTH. In a cross-sectional population study, the increase in TTH prevalence between 1989 and 2001 was associated with increased pericranial pain sensitivity, especially in women.

Bendtsen and colleagues (1996) described an abnormal, linear stimulus–response curve for pressure versus pain recorded from temporalis muscle in patients with CTTH, and a correlation with the degree of tenderness. A similar abnormality was found in patients with fibromyalgia. This qualitatively altered response could be caused by activity in low-threshold mechanosensitive (LTM) afferents, which do not normally mediate pain but have a similar linear stimulus–response function. Central sensitization after strong peripheral nociceptive input may unmask previously ineffective synapses and lead to novel effective contacts between LTM afferents and superficial dorsal horn nociceptive neurones that normally receive input from high-threshold mechanoreceptors. It was therefore considered that the qualitatively altered nociception from tender muscles in patients with chronic myofascial pain most likely reflects central sensitization of second-order nociceptors.

Myofascial trigger points are defined as a hyperirritable spots associated with a taut band in a skeletal muscle. They are painful on compression and on stretch, and usually give rise to a typical referred pain pattern. Active trigger points are a cause of clinical symptoms, (i.e. referred pain, restricted motion of the affected tissues), whereas latent trigger points may not be an immediate source of pain, but might produce other muscle dysfunctions, such as fatigue or a restricted range of motion. A recent series of pilot studies performed in a blinded fashion reported an increased number of active trigger points both in patients with frequent ETTH and in patients with CTTH. In the latter, the trigger points were positively correlated with headache severity.

Taken together, these results confirm that myogenic referred pain elicited by active trigger points in the head, neck, and shoulder muscles may contribute to head pain patterns in TTH, and that persistent peripheral sensitization in active trigger points could lead to sensitization of second-order nociceptive neurones in the spinal trigeminal nucleus.

PPTs determined with an algometer are on average decreased in CTTH, but the difference with healthy volunteers is less pronounced than for manual palpation. In ETTH, pain detection thresholds at cephalic sites are usually no different from those determined in healthy controls. PPTs in CTTH were also abnormal at extracephalic sites, for instance at the Achilles tendon, in paravertebral muscles, or in the fingers. This is yet further evidence suggesting that diffuse disruption of central pain-modulating systems is one of the pathophysiological hallmarks of CTTH. PPTs are lower in the cranium than in the extremities, and this might explain why a general lowering of pain thresholds (increased sensitivity) can result in head pain without pain in the rest of the body. Finally, the normal increase in PPTs during isometric muscular contraction is abolished over the temple in CTTH; this also favours an abnormal control of nociception in trigeminal nucleus caudalis. A similar abnormality was found in patients with fibromyalgia, but at both cephalic and extracephalic sites, which reinforces the concept that fibromyalgia and TTH may have common pathophysiological denominators.

Sensitivity to electrical stimuli is increased in cephalic and extracephalic regions (generalized hyperalgesia) in patients with CTTH, suggesting that pain processing in the central nervous system is abnormal. These studies also indicated that suprathreshold stimuli are more sensitive than pain thresholds for the evaluation of generalized pain perception.

7.2.2 Nociceptive reflexes and pathways

Brainstem reflexes are interesting non-invasive tools for investigating the central processing of sensory information from the cephalic region, whereas the flexion reflex obtained in biceps femoris muscle after electrical stimulation of the sural nerve is a spinally mediated nociceptive reflex. Both have been investigated extensively in TTH.

7.2.3 Temporalis muscle exteroceptive silent periods

Painful stimuli in the trigeminal territory induce two successive suppressions of voluntary EMG activity in jaw-closing muscles (temporalis and masseter), called ES1 and ES2, which are mediated respectively by oligosynaptic and polysynaptic interneuronal brainstem circuits. The second temporalis exteroceptive silent period (ES2) was found to be absent or reduced in patients with CTTH by some groups, leading to the hypothesis that inhibitory interneurones might be inadequately activated because of a dysfunctioning descending control from the limbic system (periaqueductal grey, amygdala, hypothalamus, and orbitofrontal cortex) via nucleus raphe magnus. In patients with ETTH, ES2 duration is normal. Although recent studies have confirmed the reduction of ES2 duration in CTTH, ES2 was found to be normal in several other studies. Carbon dioxide laser-evoked temporalis muscle suppression periods were normal in ETTH and CTTH, although in the same study electrically evoked ES2 was significantly reduced in both patients groups. Such discrepancies could be method and/or patient related, knowing that ES2 can also be influenced by psychological traits such as anxiety and aggressivity. Results of pharmacological modulations of ES2 suggest that the inhibitory interneurones mediating ES2 are inhibited by serotonergic pathways and activated by nicotinic cholinergic mechanisms; this findings is partly supported by the observation that amitriptyline, which notably blocks serotonin re-uptake, reduces ES2 in patients with CTTH.

7.2.4 **Biceps femoris flexion reflex**

A decreased threshold of the nociceptive flexion reflex as well as lower pain tolerance thresholds were found in patients with CTTH compared with controls. The slope of the stimulus intensity/visual analogue scale pain rating response curve was also steeper in CTTH. These findings might be explained by a dysfunction of endogenous antinociceptive systems, with a lowering of tone and recruitment of descending inhibitory control.

7.2.5 **Laser-evoked nociceptive cortical potentials**

Cortical potentials (P2 component) evoked by supraorbital laser-heat stimulations have an increased amplitude in CTTH, whereas heat pain thresholds are normal. This increase is proportional to the increase in the total pericranial tenderness score, and is attenuated after treatment with amitriptyline.

7.2.6 **Structural brain changes**

Using magnetic resonance imaging voxel-based morphometry, a recent study demonstrated a decrease in the volume of grey matter brain structures involved in pain processing in patients with CTTH. This decrease was positively correlated with the duration of headache, and was thought to be a consequence of central sensitization due to prolonged input from pericranial myofascial structures. Similar changes were found in patients with chronic low back pain or peripheral limb phantom pain. The precise significance of this tissue atrophy is not known, but it is tentatively attributed to excessive activation of involved structures ('overuse atrophy'). Interestingly, opposite findings (i.e. tissue density increases) have been reported in migraine.

7.3 **Neurotransmitters**

7.3.1 **Nitric oxide (NO)**

Glyceryl trinitrate (GTN), a NO donor, is able to induce an immediate headache, thought to be due to vasodilatation, and a delayed typical migraine attack in migraine subjects. In CTTH, GTN also produces an immediate headache and, after several hours, a tension-type headache comparable to that usually experienced by the patients. The immediate headache is not accompanied by a concomitant increase in pericranial tenderness, but may be associated with endogenous production of NO and sensitization of perivascular sensory afferents. This suggests that, like migraine, CTTH may be associated with central NO supersensitivity; this is supported by the reduction in headache and muscle hardness after administration of a NOS inhibitor.

7.3.2 Neuropeptides

Calcitonin gene-related peptide (CGRP) is one of the transmitters in the trigeminovascular system and its plasma levels are raised during migraine and cluster headache attacks. In CTTH, CGRP plasma levels are normal overall, irrespective of the headache state, and do not increase after GTN administration. Interictally, however, they are increased in patients with CTTH who have a pulsating quality of pain. This may suggest that the headache in certain patients who fulfil International Headache Society criteria for TTH is pathophysiologically related to migraine, if their headache has a pulsating quality.

Plasma levels of substance P, neuropeptide Y, and vasoactive intestinal peptide do not significantly differ between patients with CTTH and healthy subjects, in neither the cranial nor the peripheral circulation, and their levels are largely unrelated to the presence or absence of headache.

Serotonin (5-HT)

Results of studies on 5-HT metabolism in TTH are in part contradictory, but tend nevertheless to indicate an increased 5-HT turnover, in contrast to the findings in migraine. Interestingly, it has been shown that injectable sumatriptan, the 5-$HT_{1B/1D}$ serotonin agonist that is highly effective for acute migraine attacks, may also have significant efficacy in TTH.

7.4 Psychological studies

Emotional disturbances have been implicated as risk factors for TTH. Stress and mental tension seem to be the most common precipitating factors of TTH, and a positive correlation between headache and stress has been shown in patients with TTH. A recent review concluded that there is no increase in anxiety or depression in patients with infrequent TTH, whereas frequent TTH is associated with higher rates of anxiety and depression. As a matter of fact, it is difficult in these patients to determine whether their depressive mood is primary or secondary. Of interest for pathophysiological research, however, is the finding that depressed headache sufferers are more vulnerable to headache induced by a laboratory stressor.

7.5 Genetics

Genetic epidemiological studies of TTH in the general population or in twin pairs have indicated an increased genetic risk for CTTH and frequent ETTH, but not for infrequent ETTH. The transmission suggests complex inheritance. In a practical way, one can adopt the view that the great majority of people in the general population, perhaps all, have the potential to develop TTH if exposed to sufficiently strong environmental factors. Only a small proportion, however, will develop frequent or chronic TTH, because of a combination of external factors and anxio-depressive features, the latter probably genetically determined.

7.6 A model for TTH pathogenesis

Considering the various pathophysiological abnormalities found in TTH and their differences between TTH types, the following model can be proposed as a working hypothesis (Figure 7.1).

TTH may be the result of an interaction between changes in the descending control of second-order trigeminal brainstem nociceptors and interrelated peripheral changes, such as myofascial pain sensitivity and strain in pericranial muscles. An acute episode of ETTH may occur in many individuals who are otherwise perfectly normal. It can be brought on by physical stress, usually combined with psychological stress or non-physiological working positions. In such cases, increased nociception from strained muscles may be the primary cause of the headache, possibly favoured by a central temporary change in pain control due to stress.

Emotional mechanisms increase muscle tension via the limbic system and at the same time reduce tone in the endogenous antinociceptive system. With more frequent episodes of headache, central changes become increasingly more important. Long-term potentiation/sensitization of nociceptive neurones and decreased activity in the antinociceptive system gradually lead to CTTH. These central changes probably predominate in frequent ETTH and in CTTH. The relative importance of peripheral and central factors may, however, vary between patients and over time in the same patient. Genetic components are likely to promote the psychological and central changes leading to CTTH, whereas environmental factors are the major culprit in ETTH.

Such a model explains why TTH is related pathophysiologically to other functional pain disorders in which peripheral myofascial and central factors interact, such as fibromyalgia and regional myofascial pain.

The pathogenic model proposing that TTH and migraine are the opposite ends of a phenotypic spectrum of the same disorder is not likely to be applicable to most patients with TTH. Although it may apply to patients with migraine who also have 'tension-type like' interval headaches, a large proportion of subjects suffering from TTH never present with full-blown migraine attacks and do not respond to antimigraine treatments.

To conclude, TTH is clinically and pathophysiologically heterogeneous. With regard to pathogenesis, pericranial myofascial mechanisms are probably of importance in ETTH, whereas sensitization of pain

Figure 7.1 A model for the pathophysiology of chronic tension-type headache

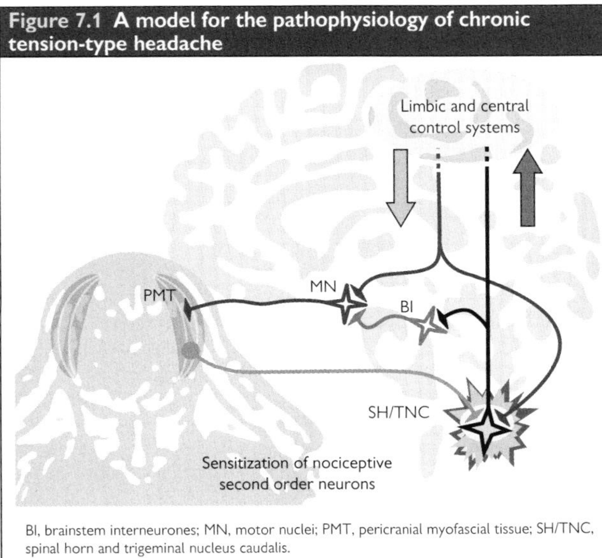

BI, brainstem interneurones; MN, motor nuclei; PMT, pericranial myofascial tissue; SH/TNC, spinal horn and trigeminal nucleus caudalis.

pathways in the central nervous system (due to prolonged nociceptive stimuli from pericranial myofascial tissues) and inadequate endogenous pain control seem to be responsible for the conversion of episodic to chronic TTH.The nociceptive input from myofascial pericranial tissues is increased for unknown reasons, resulting in plastic changes (sensitization of nociceptive second-order neurones) in the spinal dorsal horn (second and third cervical segments)/trigeminal nucleus. The nociceptive input to supraspinal structures will therefore be considerably increased, and may result in increased excitability of supraspinal neurones as well as decreased inhibition or increased facilitation of nociceptive transmission in the spinal dorsal horn/trigeminal nucleus. The central neuroplastic changes may also increase the drive to motor neurones at both the supraspinal and the segmental level, resulting in slightly increased muscle activity and increased muscle hardness.

Figure 7.1 adapted from Fumal A and Schoenen J (2008). Tension-type headache: current research and clinical management. *Lancet Neurol* **7**: 70–83, with permission from Elsevier.

Key references

Ashina M (2004). Neurobiology of chronic tension-type headache. *Cephalalgia* **24**, 161–72.

Ashina M, Bendtsen L, Jensen R, Sakai F and Olesen J (1999). Muscle hardness in patients with chronic tension-type headache: relation to actual headache state. *Pain* **79**, 201–5.

Ashina S, Bendtsen L, Ashina M, Magerl W and Jensen R (2006). Generalized hyperalgesia in patients with chronic tension-type headache. *Cephalalgia* **26**, 940–8.

Bendtsen L and Treede RD (2005). Sensitization of myofascial pain pathways in tension-type headaches. In: *The Headaches* (ed. J Olesen, PJ Goadsby, N Ramadan, P Tfelt-Hansen and KM Welch), pp 635–9. Lippincott Williams Wilkins, Philadelphia.

Bendtsen L, Jensen R and Olesen J (1996). Qualitatively altered nociception in chronic myofascial pain. *Pain* **65**, 259–64.

Bendtsen L, Fumal A and Schoenen J. Tension-type headache: mechanisms. In: *Handbook of Clinical Neurology: Headache* (ed. G Nappi and M Moskowitz) (in press).

Buchgreitz L, Lyngberg A, Bendtsen L and Jensen R (2007). Increased prevalence of tension-type headache over a 12-year period is related to increased pain sensitivity. A population study. *Cephalalgia* **27**, 145–52.

de Tommaso M, Shevel E, Pecoraro C *et al.* (2006). Intra-oral orthosis vs amitriptyline in chronic tension-type headache: a clinical and laser evoked potentials study. *Head Face Med* **2**, 15.

Fernández-de-Las-Peñas C, Simons D, Cuadrado ML and Pareja J (2007). The role of myofascial trigger points in musculoskeletal pain syndromes of the head and neck. *Curr Pain Headache Rep* **11**, 365–72.

Fumal A and Schoenen J (2008). Tension-type headache: current research and clinical management. *Lancet Neurol* **7**, 70–83.

Heckman BD and Holroyd KA (2006). Tension-type headache and psychiatric comorbidity. *Curr Pain Headache Rep* **10**, 439–47.

Janke EA, Holroyd KA and Romanek K (2004). Depression increases onset of tension-type headache following laboratory stress. *Pain* **111**, 230–8.

Miner JR, Smith SW, Moore J and Biros M (2007). Sumatriptan for the treatment of undifferentiated primary headaches in the ED. *Am J Emerg Med* **25**, 60–4.

Olesen J and Schoenen J (1999). Tension-type headache, cluster headache, and miscellaneous headaches. Synthesis of tension-type headache mechanisms. In: *The Headaches* (2nd edn) (ed. J Olesen, P Tfelt-Hansen and KMA Welch), pp 615–18. Lippincott Williams & Wilkins, New York.

Sandrini G, Rossi P, Milanov I, Serrao M, Cecchini AP and Nappi G (2006). Abnormal modulatory influence of diffuse noxious inhibitory controls in migraine and chronic tension-type headache patients. *Cephalalgia* **26**, 782–9.

Schmidt-Wilcke T, Leinisch E, Straube A *et al.* (2005). Gray matter decrease in patients with chronic tension-type headache. *Neurology* **65**, 1483–6.

Schoenen J and Bendtsen L (2006). Neurophysiology of tension-type headaches. In: *The Headaches* (3rd edn) (ed. J Olesen, PJ Goadsby, N Ramadan, P Tfelt-Hansen and KM Welch), pp 643–50. Lippincott Williams & Wilkins, Philadelphia.

Schoenen J and Wang W (1997). Tension-type headache. In: *Headache* (ed. PJ Goadsby and SJ Silberstein), pp 177–200. Butterworth-Heinemann, Boston.

Schoenen J (2004). Tension-type headache and fibromyalgia: what's common, what's different. *Neurol Sci* **25**, S157–9.

Chapter 8

Cluster and other trigeminal autonomic cephalalgias

Arne May

Key points

- Inflammation of the walls of the cavernous sinus, thought to obliterate venous outflow and thus injure the traversing sympathetic fibres of the intracranial internal carotid artery and its branches, is a controversial mechanism.
- The least common denominator is that primary cluster headache is characterized by hypothalamic activation with secondary activation of the trigeminofacial reflex, probably via a trigeminohypothalamic pathway.
- In longstanding chronic cluster headache, the headache and autonomic symptoms may be generated entirely through central mechanisms, and activation of the trigeminofacial reflex is no longer considered necessary to produce the full clinical picture.
- The pain of cluster headache and the other trigeminal autonomic cephalalgias does not arise from a primary dysfunction of the trigeminal nerve itself but is generated directly from the brain.

8.1 Introduction

Although cluster headache and related headaches are well defined from a clinical point of view and have been recognized for more than two centuries, their pathophysiology is still poorly understood. However, the last decade has seen remarkable progress made toward unravelling the pathophysiological puzzle. It is probably better to regard the condition as a hypothalamic syndrome rather than a simple headache. In doing so, the contributions of both peripheral and central structures are served and the (hypothalamic) symptoms, such as aggressiveness, sleep disturbance, restlessness, endocrine and vegetative symptoms typically encountered by many patients, are allowed for.

8.2 Neurovascular theories

The vascular theory has been superseded by the recognition that neurovascular phenomena seem to be more important. The excruciatingly severe unilateral pain is likely to be mediated by activation of the first (ophthalmic) division of the trigeminal nerve, whereas the autonomic symptoms are due to activation of the cranial parasympathetic outflow from the VIIth cranial nerve.

A controversial proposal is that inflammation of the walls of the cavernous sinus occurs on one side, obliterating venous outflow and thus injuring the traversing sympathetic fibres of the intracranial internal carotid artery and its branches.

8.3 The hypothalamus

The relapsing–remitting course, its seasonal variation, and the clocwise regularity of single attacks are characteristic and suggest an involvement of the biological clock, namely the hypothalamus, in the origin of the illness. Significantly lowered levels of plasma testosterone in male patients with cluster headache during cluster periods provided the first evidence of such an involvement in cluster headache. This was further supported by a reduced response to thyrotropin-releasing hormone and a range of other circadian irregularities that have been reported in patients with cluster headache. Melatonin, in particular, is a marker of the circadian system, and a blunted nocturnal peak melatonin level and complete loss of circadian rhythm have been reported in cluster headache. The endogenous circadian rhythm is run by an oscillator in the suprachiasmatic nuclei in the ventral hypothalamus, and is entrained to temporal environmental cues by light conditions via a retinohypothalamic pathway. Clinical observations thus suggest the hypothalamus or a closely related structure as a candidate for triggering an acute attack of cluster headache.

8.4 The trigeminofacial reflex

The least common denominator is that primary cluster headache is characterized by hypothalamic activation with secondary activation of the trigeminofacial reflex, probably via a trigeminohypothalamic pathway (Figure 8.1). In longstanding chronic cluster headache, the headache and autonomic symptoms may be generated entirely through central mechanisms, as activation of the trigeminofacial reflex is no longer considered necessary to produce the full clinical picture.

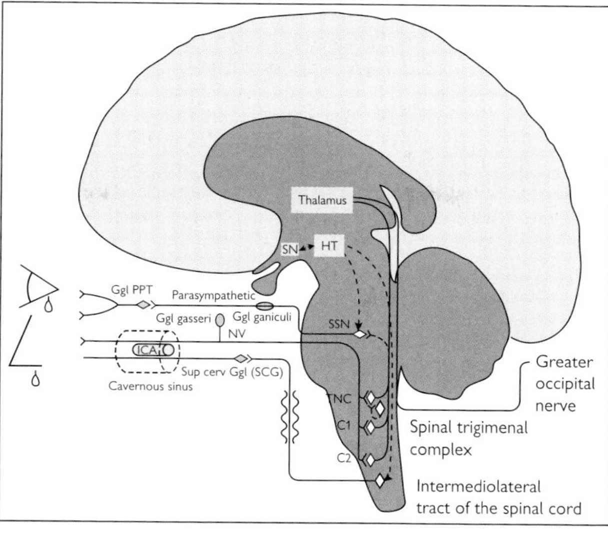

Figure 8.1 Schematic model showing most of the putative actors in the pathogenesis of cluster headache. Pain afferents from the trigeminovascular system synapse on the trigeminocervical complex (TNC), and then project to the thalamus and lead to activation in cortical areas known to be involved in pain transmission. Either a direct influence of the hypothalamus or a reflex activation of the parasympathetic outflow from the superior salivatory nucleus (SSN), predominantly through the pterygopalatine (sphenopalatine) ganglion, leads to the parasympathetic symptoms ipsilateral to the pain. A third-order sympathetic nerve lesion, thought to be caused by vascular changes in the cavernous sinus loggia with subsequent irritation of the local plexus of nerve fibres, results in a partial Horner's syndrome. The key site in the central nervous system for triggering the pain and controlling the cycling aspects is in the posterior hypothalamic grey matter region, modulated by phase-shifting in the suprachiasmatic nuclei. For details see text. Ggl, ganglion; HT, hypothalamus; ICA, internal carotid artery; NV, trigeminal nerve; PPT, pterygopalatine; SCG, superior cervical ganglion; SN, suprachiasmatic nucleus.

8.5 **Functional imaging**

Functional imaging using positron emission tomography (PET) has confirmed a highly specific activation of the hypothalamic grey in glyceryl trinitrate (GTN)-triggered and spontaneous cluster headache attacks that is involved in the pain process in a permissive or triggering manner rather than simply as a response to first-division nociception *per se*.

Figure 8.1 adapted from May A (2005). Cluster headache: pathogenesis, diagnosis and management. *Lancet* **366:** 843–55, with permission from Elsevier.

Although the headache syndromes that form the trigeminal autonomic cephalalgias (TACs), namely cluster headache, paroxysmal hemicrania, and short-lasting neuralgiform headache with conjunctival injection and tearing (SUNCT), clearly share typical clinical features; in most cases a subclassification is possible and reasonable as the therapeutical regimen and responses differ. Given that many of the basic features of SUNCT are shared by cluster headache and paroxysmal hemicrania, the question arises as to whether a shared pathophysiological basis exists that may find its visual expression in similar cerebral activation patterns.

Using functional magnetic resonance imaging and blood oxygen level-dependent (BOLD) contrast, four independent papers reporting functional imaging data in patients suffering from spontaneous SUNCT attacks all found activation next to the hypothalamic spot that was activated in cluster headache. Even in a patient suffering from excruciating trigemino-autonomic headache attacks, in whom frequency, duration, and therapeutic response allowed no clear-cut classification to one of the subtypes of trigeminal autonomic cephalgia, the same prominent activation in the hypothalamic grey matter was found. If this biological model is correct, the underlying cause for trigeminal autonomic cephalalagias may indeed be similar, and the variation in duration and frequency might be generally dependent on a different disorder of the inferior posterior hypothalamic neurones, perhaps a modulation of neuronal activity or a different involvement of the trigeminovascular system, explaining the relatively different phenotypes of these related syndromes. In any case, these studies underline the conceptual value of the term TAC for the group of headaches focusing around the trigeminal–autonomic reflex. Moreover, they emphasize the importance of the hypothalamus as a key region in the pathophysiological process of this entity.

8.6 **Orexin**

Orexin A and B (or hypocretins) are two neuropeptides synthesized by neurones located exclusively in the lateral and posterior hypothalamus, and are involved in hypothalamic regulation of autonomic and neuroendocrine functions. Orexin-containing neurones have widespread projections throughout the central nervous system, with particularly dense projections to monoaminergic and serotonergic brainstem centres.

Recently, orexins were suggested to be involved in nociception. In animal experiments they have a complex interaction with nociceptive and mechanical input, and seem to convey both decreased and enhanced nociceptive responses in the trigeminal nucleus caudalis. Interestingly, genetic analysis revealed that a specific polymorphism in the *HCRTR2* gene (receptor gene for orexins) is significantly different in patients with cluster headache and in controls, pointing to a crucial link between these peptides and cluster headaches.

8.7 Hemicrania continua

Another half-sided headache accompanied by trigeminal autonomic features is the so-called hemicrania continua. This is a strictly unilateral, continuous headache of moderate intensity, with superimposed exacerbations of severe intensity that are than accompanied by autonomic features and migrainous symptoms. The syndrome is exquisitely responsive to indometacin. Although, for theoretical reasons it is not included in the TACs, a significant activation of the contralateral posterior hypothalamus and ipsilateral dorsal rostral pons in seven patients with hemicrania continua has been described. In addition, there was activation of the ipsilateral ventrolateral midbrain that extended over the red nucleus and substantia nigra, and the bilateral pontomedullary junction. This study demonstrated nicely that the neuroimaging markers of trigeminal autonomic headaches and migrainous syndromes are demonstrated in hemicrania continua, mirroring the clinical phenotype, which in fact exhibits a certain overlap with trigeminal autonomic headaches and migraine. Taken together, just as in the case of an atypical trigemino-autonomic headache, the functional imaging data in hemicrania continua impressively emphasize that primary headache syndromes can be distinguished on a functional neuroanatomical basis by areas of activation specific to the clinical presentation.

8.8 How pathophysiology translates into treatment

Most recently, using voxel-based morphometry, a significant structural difference in grey matter density, a 'lesion' coinciding with the inferior posterior hypothalamus, was found in cluster headache but not in patients with migraine when compared to healthy volunteers. In terms of the stereotactic coordinates, this lesion was in virtually the identical area in which activation during an acute cluster headache attack was demonstrated by PET.

8.8.1 Deep brain stimulation

This work has even led to the successful introduction of a therapeutic target using deep brain stimulation of the posterior hypothalamic grey matter. Currrently, 20 patients who have undergone successful operation for intractable chronic cluster headache have been reported, some with a follow-up of more than 4 years.

When the stimulator is switched off, attacks reappear; they disappear when it is turned on again. Notably, some time elapses between turning the unipolar stimulator on or off and change in the clinical picture. The method is reversible, and the procedure is well tolerated in most patients with no relevant side-effects. However, one patient died during the operation. This led to defining operational criteria for patients who should be operated on. Of clinical interest is that hypothalamic deep brain stimulation did not result in trigeminal hypo- or anaesthesia in any of the patients treated. Neither did hypothalamic stimulation affect anaesthesia dolorosa. This observation strengthens the hypothesis that the pain of cluster headache does not arise from a primary dysfunction of the trigeminal nerve itself, but is generated directly from the brain. Electrical stimulation of the superior sagittal sinus activates the supra-optic nucleus and posterior hypothalamic area, and a monosynaptic pathway connecting the hypothalamus and trigeminal nucleus has been documented. The posterior hypothalamus is able both to decrease and to enhance nociceptive responses in the trigeminal nucleus caudalis. Little is known about the circuits and mechanisms underlying the analgesic effect of deep brain stimulation, although it probably involves activation of thalamocortical pathways and changes in cortical activity. Further research in this field is urgently needed, and the recent possibility of combining deep brain stimulation with PET will certainly help to unravel the brain circuitry implicated in stimulation-produced analgesia.

8.8.2 **Greater occipital nerve stimulation**

Patients suffering from primary headache syndromes with typically frontal symptoms, such as migraine or cluster headache, often complain of accompanying neck pain, stiffness, or tenderness, suggesting participation of trigeminal and cervical innervation in central pain-processing mechanisms in these disorders. The most likely mechanism for this observation is 'referred pain' originating from structures in the neck and projecting to facial areas, and *vice versa* at the level of second-order neurones in the brainstem, which receive convergent input from both trigeminal and cervical territories. Based on findings from experimental studies, electrical stimulation of the greater occipital nerve (GON) in animals did indeed have a facilitating effect on dural nociceptive stimulation, suggesting the subsequent induction of central sensitization on second-order neurones receiving cervical and trigeminal input. The fact that a drug-induced block of the occipital nerve inhibits the nociceptive blink reflex, and that local cortisone injection in the region of the GON has been shown to be effective in cluster headache, provides evidence for functional connectivity between cervical and trigeminal nerves in humans. Recently, occipital stimulation has been suggested as a novel therapeutic approach in refractory patients, with promising results. However, the trigeminocervical complex does not seem to be primarily facilitated in cluster headache, suggesting a more centrally located pathology of the disease. In this context it is noteworthy that with GON stimulation the time to onset of effect (up to several weeks) suggests that brain plasticity may be crucial in mediating the therapeutic effect. Further studies with longer follow-up are warranted to understand the place of invasive treatment alternatives in clinical practice.

8.8.3 **Oxygen**

Cluster headache is the only primary headache syndrome that responds to inhalation of 100% oxygen. It should be pointed out that the mechanism of the efficacy of oxygen is not understood and that none of the preventive medication is given based on a valid theoretical background, but rather a purely empirical one.

Key references

Bartsch T, Levy MJ, Knight YE and Goadsby PJ (2004). Differential modulation of nociceptive dural input to [hypocretin] orexin A and B receptor activation in the posterior hypothalamic area. *Pain* **109**, 367–78.

Cohen AS, Matharu MS and Goadsby PJ (2006). Short-lasting unilateral neuralgiform headache attacks with conjunctival injection and tearing (SUNCT) or cranial autonomic features (SUNA)—a prospective clinical study of SUNCT and SUNA. *Brain* **129**, 2746–60.

Goadsby PJ (2002). Pathophysiology of cluster headache: a trigeminal autonomic cephalgia. *Lancet Neurol* **1**, 251–7.

Goadsby PJ and Edvinsson L (1994). Human *in vivo* evidence for trigeminovascular activation in cluster headache. Neuropeptide changes and effects of acute attack therapies. *Brain* **117**, 427–34.

Goadsby PJ and Lipton RB (1997). A review of paroxysmal hemicranias, SUNCT syndrome and other short-lasting headaches with autonomic feature, including new cases. *Brain* **120**, 193–209.

Kudrow L (1987). The cyclic relationship of natural illumination to cluster period frequency. *Cephalalgia* **7**, (sup. 6), 76–8.

Leone M, Patruno G, Vescovi A and Bussone G (1990). Neuroendocrine dysfunction in cluster headache. *Cephalalgia* **10**, 235–9.

Leone M, Franzini A and Bussone G (2001). Stereotactic stimulation of posterior hypothalamic gray matter in a patient with intractable cluster headache. *N Engl J Med* **345**, 1428–9.

Matharu MS and Goadsby PJ (2002). Persistence of attacks of cluster headache after trigeminal nerve root section. *Brain* **125**, 976–84.

Matharu MS, Cohen AS, McGonigle DJ, Ward N, Frackowiak RS and Goadsby PJ (2004). Posterior hypothalamic and brainstem activation in hemicrania continua. *Headache* **44**, 747–61.

May A (2005). Cluster headache: pathogenesis, diagnosis, and management. *Lancet* **366**, 843–55.

May A and Goadsby PJ (1999). The trigeminovascular system in humans: pathophysiological implications for primary headache syndromes of the neural influences of the cerebral circulation. *J Cereb Blood Flow Metab* **19**, 115–27.

May A, Bahra A, Büchel C, Frackowiak RSJ and Goadsby PJ (1998). Hypothalamic activation in cluster headache attacks. *Lancet* **352**, 275–8.

May A, Ashburner J, Buchel C *et al.* (1999). Correlation between structural and functional changes in brain in an idiopathic headache syndrome. *Nat Med* **5**, 836–8.

Schmidt-Wilcke T, Ganssbauer S, Neuner T, Bogdahn U and May A (2008). Subtle grey matter changes between migraine patients and healthy controls. *Cephalalgia* **28**, 1–4.

Sprenger T, Valet M, Hammes M *et al.* (2004). Hypothalamic activation in trigeminal autonomic cephalgia: functional imaging of an atypical case. *Cephalalgia* **24**, 753–7.

Waldenlind E, Gustafsson SA, Ekbom K and Wetterberg L (1987). Circadian secretion of cortisol and melatonin in cluster headache during active cluster periods and remission. *J Neurol Neurosurg Psychiatry* **50**, 207–13.

Chapter 9

Secondary headaches

Hans-Christoph Diener

Key points

- Secondary headaches can be due to trauma, vascular disorder, non-vascular intracranial disorder, substance abuse or withdrawal, infection, disturbances of homeostasis, disorders of facial structures, or psychiatric disorders.
- Suspicion of secondary headaches requires cerebral imaging by computed tomography or magnetic resonance imaging.
- Headache in secondary headaches results in most cases from changes in intracranial pressure, changes in vessel diameter, or irritation of the dura. The brain parenchyma is not pain sensitive.
- Medication overuse is a frequent cause of the transition from episodic migraine or tension-type headache to chronic headache (>15 days/month).

9.1 Introduction

Headache is the leading symptom in many brain diseases (Box 9.1). Headache can be due to increased or decreased intracranial pressure or irritation of the dura. In addition, brain vessels are pain sensitive. The brain parenchyma is not pain sensitive.

9.2 Headache attributed to head and neck trauma

The pathophysiology of traumatic headache results from damage to the skull, the dura, and increased intracranial pressure. Interestingly, the persistence of headache is inversely correlated with the severity of the head trauma. Primary headaches are a risk factor for post-traumatic headache. Whiplash leads to neck pain and headache. Most patients have normal findings on radiography, computed tomography,

Box 9.1 International Headache Society classification of secondary headaches

- Headache attributed to head and neck trauma
- Headache attributed to cranial or cervical vascular disorder
- Headache attributed to non-vascular intracranial disorder and other causes
- Headache attributed to substances or their withdrawal
- Headache attributed to infection
- Headache attributed to disturbance of homeostasis
- Headache or facial pain attributed to disorder of cranium, neck, eyes, ears, nose, sinuses, teeth, mouth, or other facial or cranial structures
- Headache attributed to psychiatric disorder

of magnetic resonance imaging (MRI) of the cervical spine. Subdural haematoma causes headache due to stretching of the dura and increase in intracranial pressure.

9.3 **Headache attributed to cranial or cervical vascular disorders**

9.3.1 **Headache attributed to transient ischaemic attacks**

Transient ischaemic attacks (TIAs) and ischaemic strokes in the posterior circulation lead more often to headache than TIA in the anterior circulation.

9.3.2 **Headache attributed to subarachnoid haemorrhage**

Headache in cerebral bleeding is caused by the space-occupying effects. Subarachnoid haemorrhage leads to immediate irritation of the dura with severe headache. Ischaemia in the posterior circulation leads to headache. This is explained by the fact that the dura in the posterior fossa and in the occipital area is supplied by branches of the basilar and posterior cerebral arteries.

9.3.3 **Headache attributed to giant cell arteritis**

Headache in giant cell arteritis is due to inflammation of the vessel wall.

9.3.4 **Headache attributed to arterial dissection**

Carotid or vertebral artery pain is the leading symptom of dissections. Lesioning or stretching the vessel wall explains postendarterectomy headache and headache during carotid angioplasty.

9.3.5 **Headache attributed to cerebral venous thrombosis**

Cerebral venous thrombosis leads to irritation of the wall of the sinus or veins and via venous congestion to increased intracranial pressure.

9.4 Headache attributed to nonvascular intracranial disorder and other causes

9.4.1 **Headache attributed to high or low cerebrospinal fluid pressure**

Both increased and decreased intracranial pressure lead to headache. Headache improves in supine position with low cerebrospinal fluid (CSF) pressure and deteriorates in supine position with increased CSF pressure. Tumours cause headache via their space-occupying effect or via hydrocephalus. Meningiosis irritates the dura and might involve the Vth nerve. Hypophyseal adenoma can cause severe headache not correlated with the size of the tumour.

9.5 Headache attributed to a substance or its withdrawal

9.5.1 **Medication overuse headache**

The pathophysiology of medication overuse headache is unknown. Growing evidence shows that central sensitization may play an important role in the pathophysiology of chronicity of headache. A series of investigations using psychophysical and electrophysiological techniques clearly demonstrated a facilitation of trigeminal pain processing in patients with chronic headache. Imaging studies provide further insights into the pathophysiology of medication overuse headache. An MRI voxel-based morphometry study revealed structural brainstem changes in patients with chronic tension-type headache but not in patients with medication overuse headache. Another study investigated glucose metabolism in 16 patients with medication overuse headache before and after withdrawal, and in 68 healthy controls. The authors found reversible hypometabolic changes in brain regions belonging to the general pain network. The orbitofrontal cortex, however, showed persistent hypometabolism before and after drug withdrawal, more so when patients were overusing combination analgesics.

Psychological factors to promote medication overuse headache include the reinforcing properties of pain relief by drug consumption, a powerful component of positive conditioning. Many patients report that they take migraine drugs prophylactically because they are worried about missing work or an important social event, or they fear an imminent headache. They are often instructed by physicians or by the instructions supplied with the medication to take the migraine drug as early as possible at the start of either the aura or the headache phase of a migraine attack. Withdrawal headache is an additional factor. When the patient tries to stop or reduce the medication, the pre-existing headache worsens. Barbiturates that are contained in drugs used to treat tension-type headache have a high potential for addiction. The stimulating action of analgesics or migraine drugs and their psychotropic side-effects, such as sedation or mild euphoria, may lead to drug dependency. Barbiturates, codeine, other opioids, and caffeine are most likely to have this effect. Caffeine increases vigilance, relieves fatigue, and improves performance and mood. Patients with headache can develop physical dependence on codeine and other opioids. Although some have been on codeine for as long as 10 years, no studies have investigated the effects of codeine intake over this time period. It should be remembered that up to 10% of codeine is metabolized to morphine.

The drugs that lead to chronic medication overuse headache vary considerably in different series, depending probably on both selection of patients (e.g. 'pure' ergotamine abusers being reported) and cultural factors. Each component contained in antimigraine drugs and analgesics can potentially induce headache. This is also true for aspirin (acetylsalicylic acid) and paracetamol. It is difficult to identify a single substance, however, as 90% of patients take more than one compound at a time. Combination analgesics containing butalbital (a short-acting barbiturate), caffeine, and aspirin with or without codeine were the leading candidates for medication overuse headache. Sumatriptan can also lead to medication overuse headache. Patients who developed drug-induced headache from naratriptan and zolmitriptan have also been reported. Results from headache diaries show that patients take an average of 4.9 tablets or suppositories per day (range 0.25–25). Patients take on average 2.5 to 5.8 different pharmacological components simultaneously (range 1–14). Patients who abuse triptans take fewer doses.

One prospective study showed the characteristics of medication overuse headache. Patients who abuse analgesics develop a constant, diffuse headache of moderate intensity. They may still suffer from intermittent migraine attacks on top of the daily headache. Most patients who overuse triptans experience an increase in the frequency of migraine attacks and may experience daily migraine-like headaches. Patients who overuse ergots usually show a mixture of the two headache characteristics.

9.6 Headache attributed to infection

Meningitis leads to direct stimulation of nerve endings in the dura. Bacterial meningitis results in the production and release of mediators of inflammation (e.g. cytokines, bradykinin, and prostaglandins), which also stimulate C-fibres in the dura. The pathophysiology of headache in systemic infections with fever is unknown. Again, release of cytokines might play a role.

9.7 Headache or facial pain attributed to disorder of cranium, neck, eyes, ears, nose, sinuses, teeth, mouth, or other facial or cranial structures

Sensory organs have a rich supply of pain fibres for protective purposes (Box 9.2).

9.7.1 Cervicogenic headache

Headache in lesions of the cervical spine, in particular in cases of cervical disc prolapse, is due to convergence of C-fibre input from cervical roots on the cervical part of the nucleus caudalis of the Vth nerve.

9.7.2 Headache attributed to rhinosinusitis

The mucosa of the sinuses is richly innervated by C-fibres projecting to the nucleus of the Vth nerve.

9.7.3 Headache attributed to acute glaucoma

The mechanism of pain in glaucoma includes increased intraocular pressure, liberation of cytokines, ciliary muscle spasm, and anterior segment hypoxia.

Box 9.2 Pain-sensitive structures in the cranium

- Blood vessels
- Dura
- Sinus
- Eyes
- Ears
- Teeth
- Neck

Key references

Ayzenberg I, Obermann M, Nyhuis P *et al.* (2006). Central sensitization of the trigeminal and somatic nociceptive systems in medication overuse headache mainly involves cerebral supraspinal structures. *Cephalalgia* **26**, 1106–14.

Couch JR and Bearss C (2001). Chronic daily headache in the posttrauma syndrome: relation to extent of head injury. *Headache* **41**, 559–64.

Diener HC and Limmroth V (2004). Medication-overuse headache: a worldwide problem. *Lancet Neurol* **3**, 475–83.

Diener HC and Silberstein SD (2006). Medication overuse headaches. In: *The Headaches* (3rd edn) (ed. J Olesen, PJ Goadsby, NM Ramadan, P Tfelt-Hansen and KMA Welch), pp 971–80. Lippincott Williams & Wilkins, Philadelphia.

Fisher CM (1968). Headache in cerebrovascular disease. In: *Handbook of Clinical Neurology* (ed. PJ Vinken and GW Bruyn), pp 124–6. Elsevier, Amsterdam.

Fisher CM (1982). The headache and pain of spontaneous carotid dissection. *Headache* **22**, 60–5.

Fumal A, Laureys S, Di Clemente L *et al.* (2006). Orbitofrontal cortex involvement in chronic analgesic-overuse headache evolving from episodic migraine. *Brain* **129(Pt 2)**, 543–50.

Katsarava Z, Fritsche G, Muessig M, Diener HC and Limmroth V (2001). Clinical features of withdrawal headache following overuse of triptans and other headache drugs. *Neurology* **57**, 1694–8.

Kaube H, May A, Diener HC and Pfaffenrath V (1994). Sumatriptan misuse in daily chronic headache. *BMJ* **308**, 1573.

Keidel M, Eisentraut R, Baum B, Yagüez L and Diener HC (1993). Prospective analysis of acute headache following whiplash injury. *Cephalalgia* **13**, 177.

Levy MJ, Matharu MS, Meeran K, Powell M and Goadsby PJ (2005). The clinical characteristics of headache in patients with pituitary tumours. *Brain* **128(Pt 8)**, 1921–30.

Olesen J, Bousser M-G, Diener H *et al.* for the International Headache Society (2004). The international classification of headache disorders, 2nd edition. *Cephalalgia* **24(suppl 1)**, 1–160.

Schmidt-Wilcke T, Leinisch E, Straube A *et al.* (2005). Gray matter decrease in patients with chronic tension type headache. *Neurology* **65**, 1483–6.

Silberstein SD, Lipton RB and Dodick DW (ed.) (2007). *Wolff's Headache and Other Head Pain* (8th edn). Oxford University Press, Oxford.

Ward TN and Levin M (2005). Headache in giant cell arteritis and other arteritides. *Neurol Sci* **26(suppl 2)**, S134–7.

Part 3

Management

Chapter 10

Migraine

Carl Dahlöf

Key points

- **Diagnosis**: Taking a diagnostic history is fundamental in the management of migraine.
- **Acute symptomatic treatment**: Acute migraine management should be tailored to the needs of the individual patient, taking into account available drugs, efficacy versus side-effects, contraindications, suitability, convenience, acceptability of route of administration, and costs.
- **Prophylactic treatment**: The major objective of prophylactic therapy is to optimize the patient's ability to function normally by reducing frequency, duration, and intensity of attacks.
- **Non-pharmacological treatment**: These alternatives can be recommended as complements to pharmacotherapy.
- **Diaries and calendars**: All patients should use these tools to confirm diagnosis and follow-up of treatment.
- **Realistic aims of management**: Migraine cannot be cured, but can be managed effectively in most cases.

10.1 Diagnosis

Successful acute symptomatic and prophylactic treatment of migraine requires correct diagnosis, adequate dosage, good timing, and choice of the optimal route for drug delivery. Guidelines for the management of migraine accordingly recommend that treatment approaches be tailored to patients' individual needs. A simple seven-step approach can be used to achieve this goal (Box 10.1).

Box 10.1 Seven steps toward adequate migraine management

1. Diagnosis of migraine
2. Explaining the condition
3. Recognizing trigger factors
4. Determining type and frequency of attacks
5. Detecting co-morbid conditions
6. Introducing headache calendars
7. Initiating individualized treatment

10.2 Acute symptomatic treatment

Almost all, if not all, migraineurs take symptomatic treatment medications, either non-prescription or prescription, in an attempt to relieve the most debilitating symptoms of the migraine attack, which include pain, nausea, phonophobia, and photophobia. Studies to investigate what patients want from migraine treatment have shown that good efficacy and rapid pain relief are the attributes they value most highly. Acute migraine treatment should be tailored to the needs of the individual patient, taking into account available drugs, efficacy versus side-effects, contraindications, suitability, convenience, acceptability of route of administration, and costs.

Table 10.1 demonstrates different acute symptomatic treatment alternatives for migraine attacks. Non-specific treatments, such as aspirin, paracetamol (acetaminophen), non-steroidal anti-inflammatory drugs (NSAIDs), opiates, and combination analgesics, are used to treat a wide range of pain disorders. Specific treatments, including ergotamine, dihydroergotamine, and the triptans (selective 5-$HT_{1B/1D}$ receptor agonists), are effective for treating neurovascular headaches, such as migraine and cluster headache, but not for treating other types of pain, such as pure tension-type headache.

Triptans have become the drugs of choice when specific drugs for the acute treatment of moderate to severe attacks of migraine are needed. Sumatriptan, the first selective 5-$HT_{1B/1D}$ receptor agonist to be developed, is the most extensively studied medication in the history of migraine. Its emergence on to the market in 1991 represented the single most remarkable advance in the treatment of migraine headache. Not only did sumatriptan have a tremendous impact on patient care and clinical practice, but it generated intense pharmaceutical research and the development of a number of second-generation agents, including zolmitriptan, naratriptan, rizatriptan, almotriptan, eletriptan, and frovatriptan.

Table 10.1 Symptomatic treatment alternatives in migraine (tablet formulation and recommended dosages may vary among countries)

I First-line alternatives			
Drug	**Formulation**	**Dose**	**Maximum no. of doses/24 h**
ANALGESICS			
Aspirin	Effervescent tablet	500–1000 mg	4
Paracetamol	Effervescent tablet/suppository	500–1000 mg	4
NSAIDs			
Naproxen	Tablet/suppository	250–750 mg	2
Diclofenac	Tablet/suppository	50–100 mg	2
Ibuprofen	Tablet	400–800 mg	3
Ketoprofen	Capsules	50–100 mg	2
COMBINATION			
Paracetamol + codeine	Tablet/suppository	500–1000 mg + 30–60 mg	4
Aspirin + caffeine	Tablet	500–1000 mg + 50–100 mg	4
IIa Second-line alternatives			
Drug	**Formulation**	**Dose**	**Maximum no. of doses/24 h**
ANTIEMETICS			
Metoclopramide	Tablet/suppository	10 mg	3
Domperidone	Tablet/suppository	10–30 mg	3
PLUS			
ANALGESICS			
Aspirin	Effervescent tablet	500–1000 mg	4
Paracetamol	Effervescent tablet/ suppository	500–1000 mg	4
NSAIDs			
Naproxen	Tablet/suppository	250–750 mg	2
Diclofenac	Tablet/suppository	50–100 mg	2
Ibuprofen	Tablet	400–800 mg	3
Ketoprofen	Capsules	50–100 mg	2
OR			
COMBINATION			
Metoclopramide + aspirin	Powder	10 mg + 900 mg	3

Table 10.1 (*Contd.*)

IIb Second-line alternatives			
Drug	**Formulation**	**Dose**	**Maximum no. of doses/24 h**
TRIPTAN (5-HT$_{1B/1D}$ receptor agonists)			
Almotriptan	Tablet	12.5 mg	2
Eletriptan	Tablet	40–(80) mg	2
Naratriptan	Tablet/suppository	2.5–5 mg	2
Rizatriptan	Tablet/wafer	5–10 mg	2
Sumatriptan	Tablet	50–100 mg	2
	Nasal spray	20 mg	2
	Suppository	25 mg	2
	Subcutaneous injection	6 mg	2
Zolmitriptan	Tablet/mouth dispersible	2.5–5 mg	2
	Nasal spray	5 mg	2
ANTIEMETICS (on demand)			
Metoclopramide	Tablet/suppository	10 mg	3
Domperidone	Tablet/suppository	10–30 mg	3
III Third-line alternatives			
Drug	**Formulation**	**Dose**	**Maximum no. of doses/24 h**
ERGOT DERIVATIVES (non-selective 5-HT1B/1D agonists)			
Dihydroer-gotamine	Nasal spray	1–2 mg	2
	Tablet/suppository	0.5 mg	2
COMBINATIONS			
Ergotamine ●	Tablet/suppository	0.5–2 mg	2
caffeine		50–200 mg	
cyclizine		10–20 mg	
ANTIEMETICS (on demand)			
Metoclopramide	Tablet/suppository	10 mg	3
Domperidone	Tablet/suppository	10–30 mg	3

10.3 **Practical considerations**

The great majority of antimigraine drugs are taken by mouth and swallowed, as most patients favour this route of administration. However, the absorption after oral administration is unpredictable. During the migraine attack, the crucial gastrointestinal motility is inhibited and the gastric emptying delayed. In addition, there is always a risk that the migraine-induced nausea culminates in vomiting. As a consequence to this, the efficacy of drugs given orally to relieve migraine attacks is not consistent.

The common strategy to treat a migraine attack as soon as it begins has been used as an attempt to avoid the impaired absorption during the migraine attack. Alternatively, the clinical management of acute migraine attacks can involve the use of analgesics and NSAIDs in combination with antiemetic gastrointestinal prokinetic drugs such as metoclopramide.

In order to improve the outcome of triptan treatment, patients should be educated in the appropriate use of each of the formulations so that reliability of response can be improved.

For the majority of patients, tablets may be an appropriate choice. Although clinical trials do not demonstrate robust differences in efficacy between triptan tablets, individual patients do distinguish them and often have a preference for one triptan or dose over another.

For those having difficulties in swallowing a tablet, the freeze-dried fast-melting tablet or wafer that can be taken without water may be an option. This dosage form dissolves instantly on the tongue, and the active agent is swallowed with the saliva and absorbed from the gastrointestinal tract.

For patients who desire particularly rapid relief that cannot be provided by a tablet form, sumatriptan subcutaneous injection with a 10-min onset of action may be an appropriate choice. Patients with very severe attacks and those with vomiting may also benefit from the injection. It is noteworthy that sumatriptan subcutaneous injection should be taken after the aura to provide headache relief.

For patients with nausea who do not wish to take tablets or who fear injections, a triptan nasal spray with a 15-min onset of action or a suppository may be appropriate options. To optimize the absorption over the nasal mucosa, the nasal spray should not be taken in the supine position.

10.4 Future drugs

New antimigraine strategies that are currently under evaluation are the use of selective direct antagonists of the sensory vasoactive neuropeptides that could be released during a migraine attack. The potent vasodilator calcitonin gene-related peptide (CGRP) serves as a good example. The enriched localization of CGRP in trigeminal sensory ganglia may indicate a role in the neurogenic inflammation associated with migraine. CGRP is presently evaluated in the acute treatment of migraine, and the results of phase II studies indicate an efficacy similar to that of triptans but with better tolerability and longer duration.

10.4.1 Prophylactic treatment

The major objective of migraine prophylactic therapy is optimizing the patient's ability to function normally by reducing frequency, duration, and intensity of attacks. Preventive treatment is taken on a daily basis, whether or not the patient is having a migraine attack. In general, prophylactic drugs are indicated when patients have three or more severe migraine attacks a month and symptomatic medication use alone is not satisfactory.

Table 10.2 demonstrates the six main classes of drugs that may be used as prophylactics, including beta-blocking drugs without intrinsic sympathomimetic activity, calcium channel blockers, serotonin antagonists, NSAIDs, antiepileptic drugs, and antidepressants.

There are varying degrees of scientific evidence supporting the use of each prophylactic drug in migraine. This evidence appears to be best for propranolol, metoprolol, flunarizine, naproxen, topiramate, and amitriptyline.

The choice of preventive drug must be tailored individually, and is influenced by contraindications, potential side-effects, and the need to treat co-morbidities such as asthma, anxiety, depression, and epilepsy (Box 10.2). For example, amitriptyline can be useful in patients with a combination of tension-type headache, sleep disturbances, and migraine attacks. Flunarizine can be used to treat frequent migraine attacks in a migraineurs with asthma.

Table 10.2 Comparison of effect, adverse events, and contraindications for different classes of drugs that can be used in the preventive treatment of migraine

Class/substance	Attack frequency/ severity	Adverse effects	Contra-indications
Beta-adrenoceptor antagonists			
Propranolol	50% reduction	Bradycardia	Asthma
Metoprolol		Hypotension	Bradycardia
Atenolol		Fatigue	Cardiac failure
		Sleep disturbance	Hypoglycaemia
		Dyspepsia	
		Depression	
Calcium channel antagonists			
Flunarizine	50% reduction	Sedation	Depression
		Weight gain	Parkinson's disease
		Depression	
Verapamil		Sleep disturbance	
		Constipation	Bradycardia
		Bradycardia	Conduction defect
$5\text{-}HT_2$ antagonists			
Pizotifen	50% reduction	Increased appetite	?Narrow-angle glaucoma
Cyproheptadine		Weight gain	?Prostatic hypertrophy
		Drowsiness	
5-HT agonist			
Methysergide 💣	50–75% reduction	Nausea	Pregnancy
		Sleep disturbance	Cardiac and peripheral vascular disorders
		Peripheral vasoconstriction	Impaired kidney or liver function
		Retroperitoneal/ pleuropulmonary fibrosis	Collagen diseases

Table 10.2 (*Contd.*)			
Class/substance	**Attack frequency/ severity**	**Adverse effects**	**Contra-indications**
Antiepileptics			
Sodium valproate	50–75% reduction	Nausea,	Pregnancy
		Vomiting	Thrombo-cytopenia
		Alopecia	Liver disease
		Tremor	
		Weight gain	
Topiramate		Weight loss	
		Sedation	
		Mood changes	
		Visual disturbances	
Tricyclics			
Amitriptyline	50% reduction	Sedation	Narrow-angle glaucoma
		Weight gain	Prostatic hypertrophy
		Dry mouth	Recovery phase after myocardial infarction
		Blurred vision	
		Constipation	
		Urinary retention	
		Postural hypotension	
Non-steroidal anti-inflammatory drugs			
Naproxen	50% reduction	Heartburn	Asthma or rhinitis induced by aspirin
		Abdominal pain	Peptic ulceration
		Nausea	Severe renal impairment
		Headache	
		Tinnitus	

Box 10.2 Conditions reported to coexist with migraine

- **Neurological**: epilepsy, essential tremor, vertigo, restless legs syndrome
- **Psychiatric**: depression, anxiety, panic disorder, bipolar, Tourette's syndrome
- **Vascular**: Raynaud's phenomenon, high blood pressure (inconsistent), ischaemic stroke, subclinical stroke, white matter abnormalities, cervical artery dissection (migraine without aura)
- **Heart**: patent foramen ovale, mitral valve prolapse, atrial septal aneurysm, ischaemic cardiovascular diseases, paroxysmal supraventricular tachycardia
- **Other**: snoring/sleep apnoea, asthma/allergy, irritable bowel syndrome, systemic lupus erythematosus, non-headache pain, unfavourable risk profile (smoking, raised total cholesterol:high-density lipoprotein ratio)

It is difficult to argue that one migraine prophylactic medication is superior to another, and accordingly should be used as a first line of treatment. Therefore, the strategy to obtain physician-optimized therapy is optional. However, based primarily on documented results in controlled clinical trials and personal experience, an attempt to divide the classes of migraine preventive drugs into first-, second-, and third-line alternatives has been made (Table 10.3).

Table 10.3 Preventive treatment alternatives in migraine

Drug	Dose	No. of doses daily
FIRST-LINE ALTERNATIVES		
Atenolol	25–100 mg	1
Metoprolol	100–200 mg	1
Propranolol	40–160 mg	1
SECOND-LINE ALTERNATIVES		
Topiramate	25–50 mg	1–2
Valproate	300–500 mg	2
Flunarizine	5–10 mg	1
Amitriptyline	10–100 mg	1
THIRD-LINE ALTERNATIVES		
Methysergide	1–2 mg	2–3
ALTERNATIVES USED FOR PROPHYLAXIS BUT WITH LIMITED DATA		
Cyproheptadine	4 mg	2–4
Naproxen	250–500 mg	1–2
Pizotifen	0.5–1 mg	1–3
Verapamil	120–180 mg	2

10.5 **Practical considerations**

Preventive migraine treatment should be tailored to the individual patient. This requires that the patient understands the rationale and participates actively in decisions regarding therapeutic intervention. The patient should also be advised to fill in the headache diary, which is used when efficacy and tolerability are evaluated at follow-up visits (1–3 months later).

As a rule, patients should start on a low dose and titrate gradually up to the highest tolerable dose or, if measured, until therapeutic concentration is achieved. This is because there are substantial inter-individual differences in drug pharmacokinetics (i.e. absorption, bio-availability, metabolism, and elimination).

It appears that prophylactic drugs exert their effects slowly (over weeks), and that these also disappear more or less gradually once the treatment is stopped. Patients who are in desperate need of preventive treatment should be allowed to test class after class of preventive drugs for a couple of months until beneficial treatment effects are obtained. However, it is wise to re-evaluate the diagnosis in patients who do not respond, or who respond poorly, to all of these alternatives.

10.6 **Non-pharmacological treatment**

Treatment alternatives such as biofeedback/cognitive behavioural therapy, acupuncture, avoiding trigger factors, massage, contemplation, physiotherapy, and relaxation are usually recommended as complements to pharmacotherapy. These treatments are also the first-line treatment alternatives for adults who cannot or do not wish to take abortive or prophylactic medications. Most migraineurs have tried most of these treatments, but only cognitive behavioral therapy, acupuncture, and staying away from triggers seem to provide significant beneficial effects.

Although cure of migraine is not currently achievable, control is possible for the majority of sufferers. Reassuringly, migraine does not appear to be a progressive disorder in most patients, and migraineurs report less frequent, shorter, and/or milder attacks over time. Eventually the migraine attacks will fade away.

Further reading

D'Amico D and Lanteri-Minet M (2006). Migraine preventive therapy: selection of appropriate patients and general principles of management. *Expert Rev Neurother* **6**, 1147–57.

Goadsby PJ (2007). Recent advances in understanding migraine mechanisms, molecules and therapeutics. *Trends Mol Med* **13**, 39–44.

Holroyd KA and Drew JB (2006). Behavioral approaches to the treatment of migraine. *Semin Neurol* **26**, 199–207.

MacGregor EA (2006). Migraine and the menopause. *J Br Menopause Soc* **12**, 104–8.

Olesen J, Bousser M-G, Diener H *et al.* for the International Headache Society (2004). The international classification of headache disorders, 2nd edition. *Cephalalgia* **24(suppl 1)**, 1–160.

Olesen J, Goadsby PJ, Ramadan NM, Tfelt-Hansen P and Welch KMA (ed.) (2006). *The Headaches* (3rd edn). Lippincott Williams & Wilkins, Philadelphia.

Steiner T, Paemeliere K, Jensen R *et al.* (2007). European principles of management of common headache disorders in primary care. *J Headache Pain* **8**, S3–47.

Chapter 11

Tension-type headache

Lars Bendtsen

Key points

- Tension-type headache (TTH) is a common primary headache with tremendous socioeconomic impact.
- Non-pharmacological management is crucial, and information, reassurance, and identification of trigger factors can be effective.
- Psychological treatments with scientific evidence for efficacy include relaxation training, electromyographic biofeedback, and cognitive behavioural therapy.
- Physical therapy and acupuncture are widely used, but the scientific evidence for efficacy is sparse.
- Simple analgesics are the mainstays for treatment of episodic TTH.
- Combination analgesics, triptans, muscle relaxants, and opioids should not be used, and it is crucial to avoid frequent and excessive use of simple analgesics to prevent the development of medication overuse headache.
- The tricyclic antidepressant amitriptyline is drug of first choice for the prophylactic management of chronic TTH.
- The development of specific non-pharmacological and pharmacological managements for TTH with higher efficacy and fewer side-effects is urgently needed.

11.1 Introduction

Tension-type headache (TTH) is the most prevalent and costly headache. It is a complex disorder in which a range of heterogeneous mechanisms are likely to play a role. The treatment of the acute episode in patients with infrequent TTH is often straightforward, but in patients with frequent headaches biological mechanisms, in particular increased sensitivity of the central nervous system, as well as psychological mechanisms, often complicate the treatment. It is important to consider the mechanisms that may be important for the individual patient and to tailor the treatment accordingly.

A correct diagnosis should be assured by means of a headache diary recorded over at least 4 weeks. The diagnostic problem most often encountered is to discriminate between TTH and mild migraines. The diary may also reveal triggers and medication overuse, and will establish the baseline against which to measure the efficacy of treatments. Identification of a high intake of analgesics is essential as other treatments are largely ineffective in the presence of medication overuse. Significant co-morbidity (e.g. anxiety or depression) should be identified and treated concomitantly.

It should be explained to the patient that frequent TTH can seldom be cured, but that a meaningful improvement can be obtained with the combination of non-drug and drug treatments. These treatments are described separately below, but should go hand in hand.

11.2 Non-pharmacological management

11.2.1 Information, reassurance and identification of trigger factors

Non-drug management should be considered for all patients with TTH and is widely used. However, the scientific evidence for efficacy of most treatment modalities is sparse. The very fact that the physician takes the problem seriously may have a therapeutic effect, particularly if the patient is concerned about serious disease (e.g. brain tumour) and can be reassured by thorough examination. A detailed analysis of trigger factors should be performed, as avoidance of trigger factors may have a longlasting effect. The most frequently reported triggers for TTH are stress (mental or physical), irregular or inappropriate meals, high intake of coffee and other caffeine-containing drinks, dehydration, sleep disorders, too much or too little sleep, reduced or inappropriate physical exercise, and psychological problems, as well as variations during the female menstrual cycle and hormonal substitution. Most of triggers are self-reported and so far none of the triggers has been tested systematically.

Information about the nature of the disease is important. It can be explained that muscle pain can lead to a disturbance of the brain's pain-modulating mechanisms, so that normally innocuous stimuli are perceived as painful, with secondary perpetuation of muscle pain and risk of anxiety and depression. Moreover, it should be explained to the patient that the prognosis in the longer run is favourable, as approximately half of all individuals with frequent or chronic TTH had remission of their headaches in a 12-year epidemiological follow-up study.

11.2.2 **Psychological treatments**

A large number of psychological treatment strategies have been used to treat TTH. Three strategies have reached reasonable scientific support for effectiveness and will be described.

Relaxation training

The goal of relaxation training is to help the patient to recognize and control tension as it arises in the course of daily activities. During the training, the patient sequentially tenses and then releases specific groups of muscles throughout the body. Later stages involve relaxation by recall, association of relaxation with a cue word, and maintaining relaxation in muscles not needed for current activities.

EMG biofeedback

The aim of electromygraphic (EMG) biofeedback is to help the patient to recognize and control muscle tension by providing continuous feedback about muscle activity. Sessions typically include an adaptation phase, baseline phase, training phase in which feedback is provided, and a self-control phase where the patient practises controlling muscle tension without the aid of feedback.

Cognitive behavioural therapy

The aim of cognitive behavioural therapy (CBT) is to teach the patient to identify thoughts and beliefs that generate stress and aggravate headaches. These thoughts are then challenged, and alternative adaptive coping self-instructions are considered. A variety of exercises may be used to challenge thoughts and beliefs, including experimenting with the adoption of another person's view of the situation, actively generating other possible views of a situation, and devising a behavioural experiment to test the validity of a particular belief.

Meta-analyses have concluded that the treatments described above reduce headache by 37–50%, with no significant difference among treatments. However, the exact degree of effect is difficult to estimate because of methodological difficulties in designing appropriate placebo procedures. The most useful information on efficacy derives from a study by Holroyd *et al.* (2001) demonstrating similar improvements in patients with chronic TTH by CBT, treatment with tricyclic antidepressants, and a combination of the two treatments. All three treatment strategies reduced the headache index by approximately 30% more than placebo after 6 months. Patients who received the combination of the two treatments were more likely to show substantial reductions in TTH than those who received either treatment alone.

Although the psychological treatments seem to have similar efficacy in controlled trials, this is unlikely to be the case for the individual patient. Psychological treatments are relatively time consuming, but unfortunately there are no documented guidelines for which psychological treatment(s) to choose for the individual patient. Therefore, until scientific evidence is provided, common sense must be used. Thus, it is, for example, likely that CBT will be most beneficial for the patient in whom psychological problems or affective distress play a major role, whereas biofeedback or relaxation training may be preferable for the tense patient.

Physical therapy

Physical therapy is the most commonly used non-pharmacological treatment of TTH, and includes the improvement of posture, relaxation, exercise programmes, hot and cold packs, ultrasound and electrical stimulation, but the majority of these modalities have not been evaluated properly. Active treatment strategies are generally recommended. Spinal manipulation has no effect in episodic TTH, whereas oromandibular treatment with occlusal splints has not yet been tested in trials of reasonable quality. Thus, there is a huge contrast between the widespread use of physical therapies and the lack of robust scientific evidence for efficacy of these therapies.

Acupuncture

There are conflicting results regarding the efficacy of acupuncture for the treatment of TTH. Two recent trials found acupuncture better than no treatment, but not superior to minimal acupuncture.

11.3 **Pharmacological management**

Acute drug therapy refers to the treatment of individual attacks of headache in patients with episodic and chronic TTH. Most headaches in patients with episodic TTH are mild to moderate, and the patients often can self-manage by using simple analgesics. The efficacy of the simple analgesics tends to decrease with increasing frequency of the headaches. In patients with chronic TTH, the headaches are often associated with stress, anxiety, and depression; simple analgesics are usually ineffective and should be used with caution because of the risk of medication overuse headache with a regular intake of simple analgesics for more than 14 days a month, or triptans or combination analgesics for more than 9 days a month. Other interventions such as non-drug treatments and prophylactic pharmacotherapy should be considered. The following discussion of acute drug therapy addresses mainly the treatment of patients with episodic TTH, and the discussion of prophylactic drug therapy addresses treatment of chronic TTH.

1.3.1 Acute pharmacotherapy

imple analgesics

lost randomized placebo-controlled trials have demonstrated that spirin in doses of 500 mg and 1000 mg, and paracetamol 1000 mg, are ffective in the acute therapy of TTH. One study found no difference efficacy between solid and effervescent aspirin. There is no consis-ent difference in efficacy between aspirin and paracetamol. The non-eroidal anti-inflammatory drugs (NSAIDs), ibuprofen in doses of 00–400 mg, naproxen sodium 375–550 mg, ketoprofen 25–50 mg, nd diclofenac potassium 50–100 mg, have all been demonstrated be more effective than placebo in acute TTH. Most, but not all, omparative studies have reported that the above-mentioned NSAIDs e more effective than paracetamol and aspirin. Although simple nalgesics are effective in episodic TTH, the degree of efficacy has to e put in perspective. For example, the proportion of patients who ere pain-free 2 h after treatment with paracetamol 1000 mg, aproxen 375 mg, and placebo was 37%, 32%, and 26%, respectively. hus, efficacy is modest and there is clearly room for better acute eatment of episodic TTH.

ombination analgesics

he efficacy of simple analgesics is increased by combination with affeine 64–200 mg. There are no comparative studies examining the fficacy of combination with codeine. Combination analgesics cannot enerally be recommended because of the increased risk of medication veruse headache.

riptans and muscle relaxants

riptans have been reported to be effective for the treatment of terval headaches, which were most likely mild migraines, in patients ith migraine, but triptans do not have a clinically relevant effect in atients with episodic TTH. Muscle relaxants have not been shown be effective in episodic TTH.

onclusions

imple analgesics are the mainstays in the acute therapy of TTH Table 11.1). Paracetamol 1000 mg may be recommended as the rug of first choice because of a better gastric side-effect profile. paracetamol is not effective, ibuprofen 400 mg may be recom-nended because of a favourable gastrointestinal side-effect profile ompared with other NSAIDs. Physicians should be aware of the risk f developing medication overuse headache as a result of frequent nd excessive use of analgesics in acute therapy. Triptans, muscle elaxants, and opioids do not have a role in TTH treatment.

Table 11.1 Recommended dosages for acute and prophylactic management of tension-type headache

Acute management	Prophylactic management
Paracetamol 1000 mg	Amitriptyline 10–75 mg/day
Ibuprofen 200–400 mg	Mirtazapine 30 mg/day
Naproxen sodium 375–550 mg	
Ketoprofen 25–50 mg	
Diclofenac 50–100 mg	

Physicians should be aware of the risk of developing medication overuse headache as a result of frequent and excessive use of analgesics in acute therapy. Dosages in prophylactic management with amitriptyline are increased until efficacy or side-effects are reported.

11.3.2 Prophylactic pharmacotherapy

Prophylactic pharmacotherapy should be considered in patients with headaches for more than 15 days per month (i.e. patients with chronic TTH). For many years, the tricyclic antidepressant amitriptyline has been used. More lately other antidepressants, NSAIDs, muscle relaxants, anticonvulsants, and botulinum toxin have been tested in chronic TTH.

Amitriptyline

The tricyclic antidepressant amitriptyline is the only drug that has proven to be effective in several controlled trials in TTH. Thus, five of six placebo-controlled studies found a significant effect of amitriptyline. The two most recent studies reported that amitriptyline 75 mg/day reduced the headache index (duration x intensity) with 30% compared with placebo. The effect was longlasting (at least 6 months) and not related to the presence of depression. It is important that patients are informed that this is an antidepressant agent but has an independent action on pain. Amitriptyline should be started at low dosages (10 mg/day) and titrated by 10 mg weekly until the patient has either a good therapeutic effect or side-effects are encountered. The maintenance dose is usually 30–70 mg daily, administered 1–2 h before bedtime to help to circumvent any sedative adverse effects. A significant effect of amitriptyline may be observed already in the first week on the therapeutic dose. It is therefore advisable to change to other prophylactic therapy if the patient does not respond after 3–4 weeks on maintenance dose. The side-effects of amitriptyline include dry mouth, drowsiness, dizziness, constipation, and weight gain. Discontinuation should be attempted every 6–12 months.

Other antidepressants

The tricyclic antidepressant clomipramine and the tetracyclic antidepressants maprotiline and mianserin have been reported to be more effective than placebo, but the selective serotonin-reuptake inhibitors (SSRIs) have not been found effective. The noradrenergic and specific serotonergic antidepressant mirtazapine 30 mg/day reduced the headache index by 34% more than placebo in difficult to treat patients, including patients who had not responded to amitriptyline. The serotonin and noradrenaline reuptake inhibitor venlafaxine 150 mg/day reduced headache days from 15 to 12 per month in patients with either frequent episodic or chronic TTH. A recent study demonstrated that low-dose mirtazapine 4.5 mg/day alone or in combination with ibuprofen 400 mg/day was not effective in chronic TTH. Interestingly, ibuprofen alone increased headache, indicating a possible early onset of medication overuse headache.

Miscellaneous agents

A recent open study reported an effect for the anticonvulsant topiramate 100 mg/day. Tizanidine, botulinum toxin, propranolol or valproic acid cannot at present be recommended for the prophylactic treatment of TTH.

Conclusions

In general, the initial approach to prophylactic pharmacotherapy of chronic TTH is with the use of amitriptyline (see Table 11.1). If the patient does not respond to amitriptyline, mirtazapine could be attempted. Venlafaxine or SSRIs could be considered in patients with concomitant depression, if tricyclics or mirtazapine are not tolerated. The physician should keep in mind that the efficacy of preventive drug therapy in TTH is often modest, and that the efficacy should outweigh the side-effects.

As neither non-pharmacological nor pharmacological management is highly efficient, it is usually recommended to combine multiple strategies, although proper evidence is lacking. It is therefore reassuring that Zeeberg *et al.* (2005) reported positive results in the first study that evaluated the efficacy of a multidisciplinary headache clinic. Treatment results for all patients discharged within 1 year were evaluated. Patients with episodic TTH demonstrated a 50% reduction in frequency, 75% reduction in intensity, and 33% reduction in absence rate, whereas patients with chronic TTH responded with reductions of 32%, 30%, and 40%, respectively.

11.4 **Conclusion**

TTH is a common primary headache with a tremendous socioeconomic impact. Establishment of an accurate diagnosis is important before the initiation of any treatment. Non-pharmacological management is crucial. Information, reassurance, and identification of trigger factors may be rewarding. Psychological treatments with scientific evidence for efficacy include relaxation training, EMG biofeedback, and CBT. Physical therapy and acupuncture are widely used, but the scientific evidence for efficacy is sparse. Simple analgesics are the mainstays for treatment of episodic TTH. Combination analgesics, triptans, muscle relaxants, and opioids should not be used, and it is crucial to avoid frequent and excessive use of simple analgesics to prevent the development of medication overuse headache. The tricyclic antidepressant amitriptyline is drug of first choice for the prophylactic treatment of chronic TTH. The efficacy is modest and treatment is often hampered by side-effects. Thus, treatment of frequent TTH is often difficult, and multidisciplinary treatment strategies can be useful. The development of specific non-pharmacological and pharmacological managements for TTH with higher efficacy and fewer side-effects is urgently needed. Future studies should also examine the relative efficacy of the various treatment modalities— psychological, physical, and pharmacological treatments—and clarify how treatment programmes should be optimized to suit the individual patient.

Key references

Bendtsen L (2000). Central sensitization in tension-type headache—possible pathophysiological mechanisms. *Cephalalgia* **20**, 486–508.

Bendtsen L and Jensen R (2004). Mirtazapine is effective in the prophylactic treatment of chronic tension-type headache. *Neurology* **62**, 1706–11.

Bendtsen L and Jensen R (2006). Tension-type headache: the most common, but also the most neglected, headache disorder. *Curr Opin Neurol* **19**, 305–9.

Bendtsen L and Mathew NT (2005). Prophylactic pharmacotherapy of tension-type headache. In: *The Headaches* (ed. J Olesen, PJ Goadsby, N Ramadan, P Tfelt-Hansen and KM Welch), pp 735–41. Lippincott Williams & Wilkins, Philadelphia.

Bendtsen L, Jensen R and Olesen J (1996). A non-selective (amitriptyline), but not a selective (citalopram), serotonin reuptake inhibitor is effective in the prophylactic treatment of chronic tension-type headache. *J Neurol Neurosurg Psychiatry* **61**, 285–90.

Bendtsen L, Buchgreitz L, Ashina S and Jensen R (2007). Combination of low-dose mirtazapine and ibuprofen for prophylaxis of chronic tension-type headache. *Eur J Neurol* **14**, 187–93.

Buchgreitz L, Lyngberg A, Bendtsen L and Jensen R (2007). Increased pain sensitivity is not a risk factor but a consequence of frequent headache. A population-based follow-up study. *Pain* [Epub ahead of print].

Endres HG, Bowing G, Diener HC *et al.* (2007). Acupuncture for tension-type headache: a multicentre, sham-controlled, patient-and observer-blinded, randomised trial. *J Headache Pain* **8**, 306–14.

Holroyd KA, O'Donnell FJ, Stensland M, Lipchik GL, Cordingley GE and Carlson BW (2001). Management of chronic tension-type headache with tricyclic antidepressant medication, stress management therapy, and their combination: a randomized controlled trial. *JAMA* **285**, 2208–15.

Holroyd KA, Martin PR and Nash JM (2005). Psychological treatments of tension-type headache. In: *The Headaches* (ed. J Olesen, PJ Goadsby, N Ramadan, P Tfelt-Hansen and KM Welch), pp 711–19. Lippincott Williams & Wilkins, Philadelphia.

Jensen R and Roth JM (2005). Physiotherapy of tension-type headaches. In: *The Headaches* (ed. J Olesen, PJ Goadsby, N Ramadan, P Tfelt-Hansen and KM Welch), pp 721–26. Lippincott Williams & Wilkins, Philadelphia.

Katsarava Z and Jensen R (2007). Medication-overuse headache: where are we now? *Curr Opin Neurol* **20**, 326–30.

Lenssinck ML, Damen L, Verhagen AP, Berger MY, Passchier J and Koes BW (2004). The effectiveness of physiotherapy and manipulation in patients with tension-type headache: a systematic review. *Pain* **112**, 381–8.

Lyngberg AC, Rasmussen BK, Jorgensen T and Jensen R (2005). Prognosis of migraine and tension-type headache: a population-based follow-up study. *Neurology* **65**, 580–5.

Mathew N and Ashina M (2005). Acute pharmacotherapy of tension-type headaches. In: *The Headaches* (ed. J Olesen, PJ Goadsby, N Ramadan, P Tfelt-Hansen and KM Welch), pp 727–33. Lippincott Williams & Wilkins, Philadelphia.

Penzien DB, Rains JC, Lipchik GL and Creer TL (2004). Behavioral interventions for tension-type headache: overview of current therapies and recommendation for a self-management model for chronic headache. *Curr Pain Headache Rep* **8**, 489–99.

Steiner TJ, Lange R and Voelker M (2003). Aspirin in episodic tension-type headache: placebo-controlled dose-ranging comparison with paracetamol. *Cephalalgia* **23**, 59–66.

Stovner LJ, Hagen K, Jensen R *et al.* (2007). The global burden of headache: a documentation of headache prevalence and disability world-wide. *Cephalalgia* **27**, 193–210.

Zeeberg P, Olesen J and Jensen R (2005). Efficacy of multidisciplinary treatment in a tertiary referral headache centre. *Cephalalgia* **25**, 1159–67.

Zissis N, Harmoussi S, Vlaikidis N *et al.* (2007). A randomized, double-blind, placebo-controlled study of venlafaxine XR in out-patients with tension-type headache. *Cephalalgia* **27**, 315–24.

Chapter 12

Cluster and other trigeminal autonomic cephalalgias

Gennaro Bussone and Massimo Leone

Key points

- The first step in management is to reassure the patient that the condition is benign and to provide accurate information about it.
- There are two pharmacological approaches: acute and prophylactic.
- For cluster headache, the first choice acute treatment is the selective 5-$HT_{1B/1D}$ receptor agonist sumatriptan.
- A number of different drug options are available for prophylaxis.
- The choice of prophylactic drug is influenced by previous response, previous side-effects, contraindications, duration of symptoms, and the age and lifestyle of the patient.
- If a severe attack occurs notwithstanding prophylaxis, acute medications should be employed.
- Patients with chronic trigeminal autonomic cephalalgias who do not respond to, or have major contraindications to, prophylactic treatments may be candidates for surgical approaches.

12.1 Introduction

Patients who suffer from cluster and other trigeminal autonomic cephalgias often present to the physician in a highly anxious and agitated state, and may live in mortal fear of recurrence of an attack. The doctor's duty (after confirming or ascertaining the diagnosis) is to reassure the patient that the condition is benign and to provide accurate information about it. It is important to advise the patient to avoid triggering factors that can provoke an attack. For example, triggers for attacks during a bout of cluster headache include alcohol consumption, afternoon naps, and changes in sleep/wake rhythms.

12.2 Cluster headache

There are two pharmacological approaches to the treatment of cluster headache: prophylactic treatment and acute treatment. The aim of prophylaxis is to reduce the frequency of the attacks, both in patients with episodic cluster headache and in those with the chronic condition. In patients with episodic cluster headache, prophylaxis should be administered only during a cluster period. The older practice of continuing with prophylactic medication after a cluster period should be abandoned. The next cluster period may recur many months, or even longer, after the previous one and preventive medication—which is not without side-effects—is totally unnecessary during remission.

12.2.1 Acute treatment

To resolve an ongoing cluster headache attack, the first-choice medication is the selective 5-$HT_{1B/1D}$ receptor agonist sumatriptan (Box 12.1). Given subcutaneously, sumatriptan is effective within a few minutes. It is also available as nasal spray and 50- or 100-mg tablets. As the aim is to intervene rapidly, subcutaneous administration is preferred. However, nasal spray usually provides relief within an acceptably short period. Zolmitriptan nasal spray is also effective, but somewhat less so than sumatriptan.

Inhaled oxygen via a non-rebreathing facial mask with a flow rate of at least 7 litres per minute for about 15 min is effective for attacks of mild to moderate severity.

Nasal administration of cocaine or lidocaine (4–6%) to anaesthetize the sphenopalatine ganglion is a little used treatment for cluster headache, but may be helpful in certain cases.

12.2.2 Prophylaxis

There are various factors to weigh in the decision to begin prophylactic treatment in a patient with cluster headache, including the frequency,

Box 12.1 Treatments used for the acute treatment of cluster headache

- Triptans
  - sumatriptan, subcutaneously or intranasally
  - zolmitriptan, intranasally
- Oxygen
- Cocaine or lidocaine intranasally

duration, and severity of the attacks, patient age, and the presence of co-morbidities. One should also bear in mind that the chronic and episodic forms of cluster headache may respond differently to a given prophylactic. For episodic cluster headache it is important not to embark upon a demanding preventive regimen when the cluster period is expected will come to an end within a short period, and the headaches will disappear. Prophylactic medication is usually indicated when:

- the attacks are frequent and severe, and come to peak intensity so fast that acute treatments are ineffective
- acute treatments postpone attacks but have no effect on the course of the cluster period
- there is a tendency to overuse acute medications
- the cluster period is longlasting (several months).

The aim of prophylaxis is to bring about rapid disappearance of the attacks and to maintain an attack-free state, with minimal side-effects, until the end of the cluster period.

The principles of drug prophylaxis in episodic cluster headache are to initiate the treatment as soon as possible after the onset of a cluster period; to continue the treatments for at least 2 weeks after the disappearance of attacks; to reduce the dose gradually, not abruptly; and to restart the medication at the beginning of the next cluster period. If a severe attack occurs notwithstanding prophylaxis, acute medications such as oxygen or sumatriptan should be employed.

The choice of prophylactic drug (Box 12.2) is influenced by previous response, previous side-effects, contraindications, the duration of the cluster period, and the age and lifestyle of the patient. A combination of two or even more drugs may be necessary to terminate the attacks.

Verapamil

In recent years, calcium antagonists, and in particular verapamil, have become established for the prophylaxis of both episodic and chronic cluster headache. Verapamil is now considered the first-choice drug for cluster headache prophylaxis worldwide, although it is associated with the side-effects of constipation and sometimes hypotension. Before administering verapamil, the patient should undergo electrocardiography (ECG) to rule out severe atrioventricular conduction effects.

In a trial of verapamil 360 mg three times daily versus lithium carbonate 900 mg per day in patients with chronic cluster headache, verapamil had an efficacy greater than 75% in 80% of the patients. It was also effective more rapidly than lithium in that, in the first week of treatment, 50% of patients on verapamil improved, compared with 37% on lithium.

Box 12.2 Drugs for the prophylaxis of cluster headache

- Verapamil
- Lithium
- Corticosteroids
- Methysergide
- Clonidine
- Melatonin
- Valproate
- Topiramate

Doses of 960 mg or more daily, should only be given under specialist supervision and with regular ECG monitoring.

Lithium

Lithium at 900–1200 mg/day, which was the first-choice medication before the advent of verapamil, remains a valid alternative, particularly for chronic cluster headache. Before giving lithium, liver, kidney, and thyroid function should be checked, and during administration blood lithium levels should be kept below 1.2 mEq/l to avoid side-effects such as polyuria, tremor, vomiting, diarrhoea, oedema, and somnolence. Plasma levels of lithium sufficient to stop cluster headaches are generally below those giving rise to side-effects.

Corticosteroids

Prednisone is effective against cluster headache, particularly the chronic form, but is usually employed only in selected patients who have proved resistant to other drugs. Prednisone can be used with lithium or verapamil, but because of its side-effects is contraindicated for prolonged treatment. In patients with chronic cluster headaches, therefore, cycles lasting for 2 weeks are recommended, starting with 50–60 mg/day orally and tapering slowly to zero.

Use of intravenous cortisone should be restricted to patients refractory to all other medications and who experience daily attacks. Such patients should be hospitalized to monitor the treatment efficacy and side-effects.

Dexamethasone (8 mg/day for 1 week followed by 4 mg/day for a further week) should also be considered.

More prolonged steroid administration may be necessary in particularly refractory cases, and one should be aware of the possible long-term (in some cases irreversible) consequences of such treatments.

Methysergide

Methysergide at 4–5 mg/day is particularly effective against episodic cluster headache in young patients. As this drug is an ergotamine derivative (with major vasoconstrictive effects), the patient must be advised that it should never be taken at the same time as sumatriptan, in view of a possible synergic effect on vasospasm.

The most serious side-effect of ergotamine derivatives is retroperitoneal, pleural, and heart valve fibrosis. The risk of such effects is low if doses are kept low, but after 4–6 months of treatment the patient should be examined for renal function and assessed for cardiac disease. Abdominal ultrasonography, thoracic radiography, and magnetic resonance imaging should be considered.

Clonidine

Transdermal clonidine may be useful against chronic cluster headache; however, a recent study found it was poorly effective in the prophylaxis of episodic cluster headache.

Melatonin

In a double-blind study versus placebo, melatonin 10 mg/day showed some efficacy against episodic cluster headache. Of the ten patients treated, five experienced a clear reduction in attacks. The rationale for the use of melatonin in cluster headache derives from the fact that nocturnal levels of this substance are low in the cluster period. It is unclear, however, whether the beneficial effect is due to the fact that melatonin can improve the quality of sleep. Melatonin is perhaps best considered as an add-on therapy.

Antiepileptics

Valproate

Although a clinical study reported that valproate was effective against cluster headache, few other studies have been performed. A double-blind placebo-controlled study of sodium valproate (1000–2000 mg/day) as a preventive in cluster headache found no significant difference between patient and placebo groups. Interest in the use of this antiepileptic in the prophylaxis of cluster headache had recently been rekindled by the finding in animals that valproate prevents plasma protein extravasation from the trigeminovascular system—an effect also exercised by sumatriptan and other triptans.

Topiramate

In a study on ten patients, topiramate appeared useful in preventing cluster headache attacks. The authors' group therefore sought to investigate this drug further in an open study of 36 patients with episodic and chronic cluster headache. Of the 33 patients who completed the study, ten had chronic cluster headache and 23 had episodic cluster headache. Seven patients responded; six of these had an episodic and one a chronic form. Six of these responders received 100 mg/day and one received 150 mg/day during the treatment period. The results did not support initial expectations of efficacy, and topiramate appears to be of little use as a cluster headache prophylactic.

12.2.3 Surgical treatment of drug-resistant chronic cluster headache

About 10% of patients with chronic cluster headache do not respond, or have major contraindications, to prophylactic treatments. Such patients may be candidates for surgical approaches. It is important, however, that any proposed surgical approach should have demonstrated efficacy in ample numbers of patients. Furthermore, surgery is indicated only in patients who are unresponsive to all appropriate pharmaceutical treatments. Patient selection for surgical procedures is a difficult task. The physician should have extensive knowledge and experience of chronic cluster headache, a close professional relationship with the patient, and be prepared to dedicate time to test all possible medications and ascertain that they are ineffective. The following criteria for selecting patients for surgery should be adhered to:

- Complete inefficacy of, or major contraindications to, all appropriate prophylactic medications for cluster headache
- Chronic headache for some time (about 2 years)
- Frequent attacks (daily or almost daily)
- Strictly unilateral headache
- Normal psychological profile
- No medical conditions contraindicating deep brain stimulation.

Numerous surgical procedures have been used in the past; those to trigeminal structures, including injection of glycerol or local anaesthetics, rhizotomy, and microvascular decompression, have generally provided the best results, although corneal damage and anaesthesia dolorosa are severe—and not rare—side-effects. Although pain is reduced or disappears in about 50% of patients, a high proportion experience a recurrence of pain attacks within a year of the operation. Nevertheless, the evidence for these procedures is very scarce and should be restricted to patients who are absolutely refractory. Promising results are accumulating for the less invasive greater occipital nerve blockade, as well as bilateral nerve stimulation of the greater occipital nerve, and these procedures should always be considered before other surgical procedures.

12.2.4 Hypothalamic stimulation

The discovery of the hypothalamic activation provided support for therapeutic intervention. The authors' group proposed the use of electrode implant and stimulation to the inferior posterior hypothalamus in patients with severe intractable chronic cluster headache. The rationale was that stimulation to this area might inhibit the activation that positron emission tomography had revealed. The technique of deep brain stimulation is already widely employed to control intractable movement disorders, and experience accumulated over a decade or more has shown it to be safe and associated with few side-effects; it has the additional advantage of being completely reversible.

Twenty-four hypothalamic implants have now been performed by the authors' group on patients with chronic cluster headache, with extremely encouraging results, although less positive results and one fatal event with haemorrhagic complication have been reported.

These outcomes show that hypothalamic stimulation should be reserved for completely drug-resistant forms of chronic cluster headache, and that further experience should be collected.

12.3 Treatment of other trigeminal autonomic cephalalgias

12.3.1 Chronic paroxysmal hemicrania

Although there is no acute treatment, elective treatment with indometacin is highly effective. Doses of 150 mg/day are recommended, although lower doses may sometime be effective; higher doses are rarely necessary. Moderate efficacy has been shown with verapamil. Hemicrania continua is a similar condition to paroxysmal hemicrania, but is not considered a trigeminal autonomic cephalalgia: it too is highly sensitive to indometacin.

12.3.2 SUNCT

Short-lasting unilateral neuralgiform headache attacks with conjunctival injection and tearing (SUNCT) is a trigeminal autonomic cephalalgia that at one time was considered totally resistant to pharmacological treatment. However, recent studies have shown that lamotrigine is effective in some patients with SUNCT.

Hypothalamic stimulation might also be useful in SUNCT, but so far only a single case with an excellent result has been published.

12.3.3 Cluster-tic syndrome

In this syndrome, attacks of cluster headache and trigeminal neuralgia occur in the same patient. Usually the attacks occur at different times, but sometimes they occur together. Treatment needs to be specific for each condition (cluster headache and trigeminal neuralgia), even when they occur together.

Key references

Burns B, Watkins L and Goadsby PJ (2007). Treatment of medically intractable cluster headache by occipital nerve stimulation: long-term follow-up of eight patients. *Lancet* **369**, 1099–106.

Bussone G, Boiardi A, Merati B, Crenna P and Picco A (1979). Chronic cluster headache: response to lithium treatment. *J Neurol* **221**, 181–5.

Bussone G, Leone M, Peccarisi C *et al.* (1990). Double blind comparison of lithium and verapamil in cluster headache prophylaxis. *Headache* **30**, 411–17.

Cittadini E, May A, Strambe A, Eversd S, Bussone G and Goadsby PJ (2006). Effectiveness of intranasal zolmitriptan in acute cluster headache: a randomized, placebo-controlled, double-blind crossover study. *Arch Neurol* **63**, 1537–42.

D'Andrea G, Granella F, Ghiotto N and Nappi G (2001). Lamotrigine in the treatment of SUNCT syndrome. *Neurology* **57**, 1723–5.

El-Amrani M, Massion H and Bousser M (2002). A negative trial of sodium valproate in cluster headache: methodological issue. *Cephalalgia* **22**, 205–8.

Graham JR, Suby HI, LeCompte PR and Sadowsky NL (1966). Fibrotic disorders associated with methysergide therapy for headache. *N Engl J Med* **17**, 359–68.

Klimek A (1987). Cluster-tic syndrome. *Cephalalgia* **7**, 161–2.

Leone M (2006). Deep brain stimulation in headache. *Lancet Neurol* **5**, 873–7.

Leone M, D'Amico D, Moschiano F, Fraschini F and Bussone G (1996). Melatonin versus placebo in the prophylaxis of cluster headache: a double-blind pilot study with parallel groups. *Cephalalgia* **16**, 494–6.

Leone M, D'Amico D, Frediani F *et al.* (2000). Verapamil in the prophylaxis of episodic cluster headache: a double-blind study versus placebo. *Neurology* **54**, 1382–5.

Leone M, May A, Franzini A *et al.* (2004). Deep brain stimulation for intractable chronic cluster headache: proposals for patient selection. *Cephalalgia* **24**, 934–7.

Leone M, Franzini A, D'Andrea G, Broggi G, Casucci G and Bussone G (2005). Deep brain stimulation to relieve drug-resistant SUNCT. *Ann Neurol* **57**, 924–7.

Leone M, Franzini A, Broggi G and Bussone G (2006). Hypothalamic stimulation for intractable cluster headache: long-term experience. *Neurology* **67**, 150–2.

May A, Leone M, Áfra J *et al.* (2006). EFNS guideline on the treatment of cluster headache and other trigemino-autonomic cephalgias. *Eur J Neurol* **13**, 066–77.

Chapter 13
Secondary headaches

Zaza Katsarava and Kasja Rabe

Key points

- Correct and effective treatment of symptomatic headaches is based on an accurate diagnosis.
- Controlled randomized trials supporting therapy of symptomatic headaches are lacking.
- Intake of pain medication should be guided by the physician to prevent medication overuse headache.
- Treatment of choice for medication overuse headache is abrupt withdrawal of drugs. Prophylactic therapy might be considered in all patients at risk of medication overuse.

13.1 Introduction

To allow a differentiated management of secondary headaches, an exact medical history and appropriate further investigations are essential preconditions. As a result of the numerous different causes of secondary headaches and equally variable pathophysiology, knowledge of different therapeutic strategies is indispensable.

13.2 Headache attributed to head and neck trauma

Headache as part of the acute postconcussion syndrome is treated with acute pain medications. In migrainous exacerbation of post-traumatic headache, triptans could be used. In chronic post-traumatic headache, repetitive intravenous dihydroergotamine was described to be effective, but evidence is lacking. As regular intake of drugs for acute headache carries a risk for developing medication overuse headache, preventive treatment is a very important part of the therapeutic strategy. Antidepressants can be used as preventive therapy, as was shown by Tyler *et al.* for various different post-traumatic headaches. However, these findings could not be confirmed in a trial by

Saran. Behaviour modification, biofeedback, counselling, physical exercise, massage, and psychotherapy were shown to improve the medical condition. The treatment can be extended to cold, heat, and electrotherapy.

13.3 Headache attributed to cranial or cervical vascular disorders

13.3.1 Headache attributed to transient ischaemic attacks

Because patients with transient ischaemic attacks (TIAs) or ischaemic strokes receive medication with platelet inhibitors for stroke prophylaxis, the accompanying headache should be managed with paracetamol, which does not interact with the coagulation system.

Dipyridamole taken after the stroke for secondary stroke prevention might result in delayed headache. In patients with pre-existing migraine, dipyridamole-induced headache is observed more often. To avoid this undesirable side-effect, reduction of the usual dose can be attempted. The headache side-effects of dipyridamole usually settle within a few days. Clopidogrel is an alternative option.

If headache evolves after thrombolysis, cerebral computed tomography must be performed immediately to rule out intracranial haemorrhage.

13.3.2 Headache attributed to subarachnoid haemorrhage

Headache occurring in patients with subarachnoid haemorrhage should be treated with paracetamol or codeine. Only when symptoms do not resolve should stronger opioids be used. The dose should be as low as possible to avoid reducing the level of consciousness and complicating clinical assessment of the patient.

13.3.3 Headache attributed to giant cell arteritis

In patients with suspected giant cell arteritis, treatment with oral corticosteroids should be started as soon as possible. A higher dose of corticosteroids (up to 120 mg prednisolone) or intravenous administration (up to 1000 mg methylprednisolone) might be chosen in patients with an acute neurological syndrome or rapidly worsening neurological status. Thereafter, the medication should be tapered slowly in 2.5–5-mg reductions every 1–3 weeks. Most patients will require prednisolone for up to 2 years. Other immunosuppressant drugs have not shown consistent effectiveness.

The headache is expected to improve within a few days after initiation of treatment, but might persist for 2–4 weeks. The erythrocyte sedimentation rate may become normal within 1–2 weeks, and can be used to monitor treatment success.

13.3.4 **Headache attributed to arterial dissection**

Headache due to arterial dissection should be treated with medications without a procoagulant or vasoconstriction effect, for example paracetamol or opioids.

13.3.5 **Headache attributed to cerebral venous thrombosis**

Headache is often a leading symptom of cerebral venous thrombosis. In this case, anticoagulation is the treatment of choice and symptomatic management of the headache should include only medication without a procoagulant effect (e.g. paracetamol or aspirin).

13.4 **Headache attributed to non-vascular intracranial disorder and other causes**

13.4.1 **Headache attributed to high/low cerebrospinal fluid pressure**

Intracranial high cerebrospinal fluid (CSF) pressure might be idiopathic or due to secondary causes. Treatment strategy for idiopathic intracranial hypertension includes lowering the intracranial pressure through repeated lumbar punctures and diuretics. The carbonic anhydrase inhibitor acetazolamide reduces CSF production and seems to be effective, but prospective trials are lacking. Initially, acetazolamide is given twice daily with a dose of 500 mg daily, and gradually increased thereafter. Under close monitoring of electrolytes, it can be combined with furosemide. Topiramate has some effects due to carbonic anhydrase inhibition, and loss of weight may be a side-effect. For acute treatment, symptomatic medication as paracetamol, aspirin, or ibuprofen is given. An important aim is to lose weight.

The treatment of headache attributed to low CSF pressure due to CSF leaks has not been investigated in trials. Management includes epidural blood patch, epidural infusion of dextran, surgical repair, bed rest, increased fluid intake, caffeine, theophylline, and steroids. Spontaneous recovery is observed in several patients, but a minority continue with clear orthostatic headache. Headache after lumbar puncture is observed quite frequently and resolves mostly spontaneously. Patients should stay in bed if suffering from severe symptoms. If necessary, caffeine and/or blood patch treatment can be prescribed, also after several months' delay.

13.5 Headache attributed to substance or its withdrawal

13.5.1 Medication overuse headache

Medication overuse headache is a reason for failure of prophylactic medication, hence early diagnosis is important. Patients should record their present and prior use of medication, they should keep a headache diary for at least 1 month to record the frequency of headache and drug use. The treatment of choice is complete withdrawal of acute headache medication. Ergots, triptans, and non-opioid drugs should be stopped abruptly. Opioids and barbiturates should be withdrawn more slowly, depending on the dose and duration of intake. Discontinuation of overuse resulted in a mean reduction of headache frequency of between 18% (tension-type headache) and 51% (migraine). Rossi *et al.* (2006) reported effective withdrawal in 75% of transformed migraine patients with low medical needs.

There is no definite consensus regarding whether to arrange the withdrawal as an inpatient or outpatient. In patients with expected difficulties (unsuccessful self-withdrawals beforehand, medication overuse headache for several years, concomitant depression or anxiety disorder, insufficient family support, intake of psychotropic drugs or codeine), inpatient withdrawal is favoured. Educating the patient and their family about the disease is most important. Suhr *et al.* (1999) showed that outpatient and inpatient settings can provide the same results, if sufficient advice is given. The results were confirmed by an Italian trial, but restricted to patients without previous detoxification treatments, coexisting psychiatric illnesses, or who were taking opioids, benzodiazepines, or barbiturates.

Abrupt withdrawal can lead to withdrawal headache, usually lasting from 2 to 10 days (average 3.5 days), which can be accompanied by nausea, vomiting, arterial hypotension, tachycardia, sleep disturbances, restlessness, anxiety, and nervousness. Even in patients using barbiturate-containing drugs, hallucinations or seizures are occasionally observed. Patients taking only triptans have a shorter withdrawal than patients overusing ergots or analgesics. Within the withdrawal phase, patients should try to avoid acute pain medication. If this is not possible, the medication used should not be that which was taken during overuse. Several strategies have been suggested for treatment of withdrawal headache and concomitant symptoms, including treatment with naproxen, aspirin, intravenous dihydroergotamine, sumatriptan, or prednisone. Studies of the management of withdrawal headache with prednisone have given mixed results. Krymchantowski and Barbosa (2000) found that prednisone (prednisolone) effectively reduced withdrawal symptoms, including rebound headache. Supporting data were reported by Pageler *et al.* (2008) in a small placebo-controlled study. A recent Norwegian placebo-controlled trial had negative findings. In patients with nausea, metoclopramide or domperidone can be prescribed. Fluids can be replaced intravenously. If agitation is observed, doxepine can be prescribed. Symptoms of opioid withdrawal should be treated with clonidine.

Patients need the support of treating physicians and nurses, as well as encouragement from family and friends. Behavioural techniques such as relaxation therapy and stress management should be initiated as soon as the withdrawal symptoms fade.

The preventive treatment strategy varies between centres, and evidence-based consensus is still lacking. Although a recent study reported that only 47% of patients were in need for medical prophylaxis after 2 months' detoxification, most centres recommend early preventive treatment, started immediately during withdrawal and depending on the type of the primary headache. Although most prophylactic drugs are ineffective in patients with medication overuse headache, clinical trials suggest that valproic acid and topiramate may have some benefit in reducing daily headaches in these patients. In patients with migraine, beta-blockers might additionally improve withdrawal symptoms. In patients with chronic tension headache, tricyclic antidepressants can be prescribed. Patients often respond to prophylactic medication that was ineffective before withdrawal. Education of patients is very important in preventing relapse. Patients should be reviewed by a neurologist or psychologist for at least the first year. With help of a headache diary, frequency of headache and medication intake should be recorded. Patients should be urged to restrict medication intake.

13.6 Headache attributed to infection

Patients with headache attributed to intracranial infection should be managed with antibiotics, corticosteroids, and symptomatic acute medication, such as paracetamol, aspirin, or ibuprofen.

13.7 Headache or facial pain attributed to disorder of the cranium, neck, eyes, ears, nose, sinuses, teeth, mouth, or other facial or cranial structures

13.7.1 Cervicogenic headache

For effective treatment of cervicogenic headache, a multimodal concept, including pharmacological, physical, and surgical methods, should be pursued. At present, there is no proven therapy for cervicogenic headache. Non-steroidal anti-inflammatory drugs (NSAIDs), tricyclic antidepressants, and muscle relaxants are used frequently. Pharmacological agents should be applied in sufficient dosage and for a sufficiently long duration to judge their effectiveness. The effect of therapy should be recorded in a headache diary. Treatment might start with a NSAID such as aspirin, diclofenac, ibuprofen, or naproxen. If necessary, an anti-ulcer drug should be prescribed. Other options include paracetamol and metamizole . For gastrointestinal side-effects, cyclo-oxygenase 2-selective NSAIDs can be used. In patients with an increase of muscle tonus, muscle relaxants might be helpful. To prevent medication overuse headache, the dosage and duration of treatment should be restricted. If treatment is ineffective or improvement slow, management with tricyclic antidepressants can be tried. Further prophylactic therapy includes valproic acid, gabapentin, or pregabalin.

Various other treatments have been tried (infliximab, botulinum toxin, transcutaneous electrical nerve stimulation), but have not been proven to be effective in controlled trials.

Jull and colleagues (2002) showed that treatment with manual therapy and/or exercise was more effective at reducing the frequency and intensity of headache than no specific treatment. Slowly progressive muscle stretching and cervical manual traction should be favoured.

In 1995, Pikus and Phillips presented a study in which patients, who obtained relief of headache from diagnostic blockage of the C2 spinal nerve, improved after decompression and microsurgical neurolysis of the C2 spinal nerve. A different approach was reported by Slipman *et al.* (2001), who injected steroids into the C2–C3 zygapophyseal joint. If diagnostic block into the C2–C3 zygapophyseal joint shows relief of symptoms, denervation of the joint by radiofrequency neurotomy of the third occipital joint could be performed. However, there is no scientific evidence to support the effectiveness of this procedure.

Anaesthetic blocks of C2, or of the major occipital nerve, can be tried when pharmacological and manual/physical therapy fail. Currently, surgical interventions cannot be recommended owing to the shortcomings of previous trials and the lack of persistent improvement.

13.7.2 **Headache attributed to rhinosinusitis**

In otherwise healthy patients, acute rhinosinusitis does not usually require antibiotic treatment because it is typically caused by a virus. If symptoms continue for more than 10–14 days, bacterial rhinosinusitis is assumed to be present, and should be treated with a broad-spectrum oral antibiotic for 10–14 days. Swollen nasal mucosa should be alleviated by locally active vasoconstrictor agents, but only for 3 days. If prolonged treatment is necessary, oral decongestants can be prescribed. To prevent crusting of secretions and to facilitate mucociliary clearance, steam and saline can be used. Persistent symptoms r recurrent infections should be further evaluated by means of euroimaging or endoscopy, and, if necessary, treated surgically. Sinus ampling for culture can be attempted and antibiotics adapted.

3.7.3 Headache attributed to acute glaucoma

or correct treatment of acute glaucoma, a rapid diagnosis and referral o an ophthalmologist is necessary. Therapy includes miotics, aceta-olamide, mannitol and beta-blockers.

Key references

Boe MG, Mygland A and Salvesen R (2007). Prednisolone does not reduce withdrawal headache: a randomized, double-blind study. *Neurology* **69**, 26–31.

ritsche G, Eberl A, Katsarava Z, Limmroth V and Diener HC (2001). Drug-induced headache: long-term follow-up of withdrawal therapy and persistence of drug misuse. *Eur Neurol* **45**, 229–35.

ull G, Trott P, Potter H *et al.* (2002). A randomized controlled trial of exercise and manipulative therapy for cervicogenic headache. *Spine* **27**, 1835–43.

Katsarava Z, Fritsche G, Muessig M, Diener HC and Limmroth V (2001). Clinical features of withdrawal headache following overuse of triptans and other headache drugs. *Neurology* **57**, 1694–8.

Katsarava Z, Muessig M, Dzagnidze A, Fritsche G, Diener HC and Limmroth V (2005). Medication overuse headache: rates and predictors for relapse in a 4-year prospective study. *Cephalalgia* **25**, 12–15.

Kruuse C, Lassen LH, Iversen HK, Oestergaard S and Olesen J (2006). Dipyridamole may induce migraine in patients with migraine without aura. *Cephalalgia* **26**, 925–33.

Krymchantowski AV and Barbosa JS (2000). Prednisone as initial treatment of analgesic-induced daily headache. *Cephalalgia* **20**, 107–13.

Martelletti P and Van Suijlekom H (2004). Cervicogenic headache. Practical approaches to therapy. *CNS Drugs* **18**, 793–805.

McDonald GJ, Lord SM and Bogduk N (1999). Long-term follow up of patients treated with cervical radiofrequency neurotomy for chronic neck pain. *Neurosurgery* **45**, 61.

Mei D, Ferraro D, Zelano G *et al.* (2006). Topiramate and triptans revert chronic migraine with medication overuse to episodic migraine. *Clin Neuropharmacol* **29**, 269–75.

Pageler L, Katsarava Z, Diener HC and Limmroth V (2008). Prednisone vs. placebo in withdrawal therapy following medication overuse headache. *Cephalalgia* **28**, 152–6.

Pikus HJ, Phillips JM (1995). Characteristics of patients successfully treated for cervicogenic headache by surgical decompression of the second cervical root. *Headache* **35**, 621–9.

Pini LA, Cicero AF and Sandrini M (2001). Long-term follow-up of patients treated for chronic headache with analgesic overuse. *Cephalalgia* **21**, 878–83.

Relja G, Granato A, Bratina A, Antonello RM and Zorzon M (2006). Outcome of medication overuse headache after abrupt inpatient withdrawal. *Cephalalgia* **26**, 589–95.

Rossi P, Di Lorenzo C, Faroni J, Cesarino F and Nappi G (2006). Advice alone vs. structured detoxification programmes for medication overuse headache: a prospective, randomized, open-label trial in transformed migraine patients with low medical needs. *Cephalalgia* **26**, 1097–105.

Schoeman JF (1994). Childhood pseudotumor cerebri: clinical and intracranial pressure response to acetazolamide and furosemid treatment in a case series. *J Child Neurol* **9**, 130–4.

Slipman CW, Lipetz JS, Plastaras CT, Jackson HB, Yang ST and Meyer AM (2001). Therapeutic zygapophyseal joint injections for headaches emanating from the C2–3 joint. *Am J Phys Med Rehabil* **80**, 182–8.

Suhr B, Evers S, Bauer B, Gralow I, Grotemeyer KH and Husstedt IW (1999). Drug-induced headache: long-term results of stationary versus ambulatory withdrawal therapy. *Cephalalgia* **19**, 44–9.

Tribl GG, Schnider P, Wober C *et al.* (2001). Are there predictive factors for long-term outcome after withdrawal in drug-induced chronic daily headache? *Cephalalgia* **21**, 691–6.

Tyler GS, McNeely HE, Dick ML (1980). Treatment of post-traumatic headache with amitriptyline. *Headache* **20**, 213–6.

Vakharia SB, Thomas PS, Rosenbaum AE, Wasenko JJ and Fellows DG (1997). Magnetic resonance imaging of cerebrospinal fluid leak and tamponade effect of blood patch in postdural puncture headache. *Anesth Analg* **84**, 585–90.

Zeeberg P, Olesen J and Jensen R (2005). Efficacy of multidisciplinary treatment in a tertiary referral headache centre. *Cephalalgia* **25**, 1159–67.

Index

T

V

W

Z